LIFT YOUR VIBE

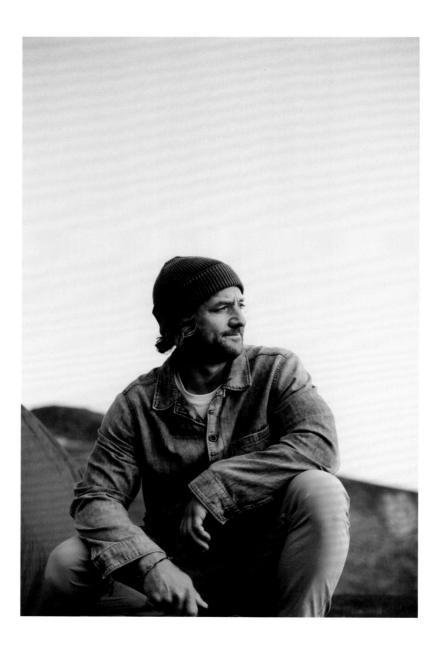

LIFT YOUR VIBE

Eat, breathe and flow to sleep better,
find peace and live your best life

Richie Norton

With photography by Issy Croker

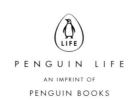

PENGUIN LIFE

AN IMPRINT OF

PENGUIN BOOKS

PENGUIN LIFE

UK | USA | Canada | Ireland | Australia
India | New Zealand | South Africa

Penguin Life is part of the Penguin Random House group of companies
whose addresses can be found at global.penguinrandomhouse.com.

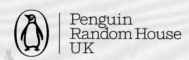

Penguin
Random House
UK

First published 2021
001

Colour reproduction by Altaimage Ltd
Printed and bound in China by C&C Offset Printing Co., Ltd

The authorized representative in the EEA is Penguin Random House Ireland,
Morrison Chambers, 32 Nassau Street, Dublin D02 YH68

A CIP catalogue record for this book is available from the British Library

ISBN: 978–0–241–44869–4

www.greenpenguin.co.uk

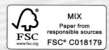

MIX
Paper from
responsible sources
FSC® C018179

Penguin Random House is committed to a
sustainable future for our business, our readers
and our planet. This book is made from Forest
Stewardship Council® certified paper.

Dedicated to my mum and dad,
and all my teachers who have been
part of this ride so far

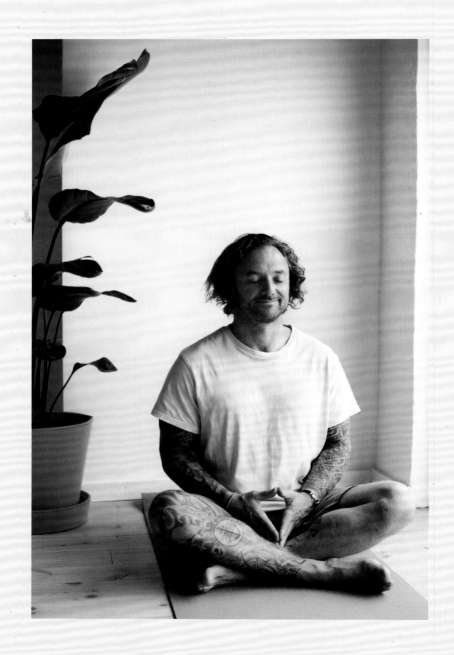

Contents

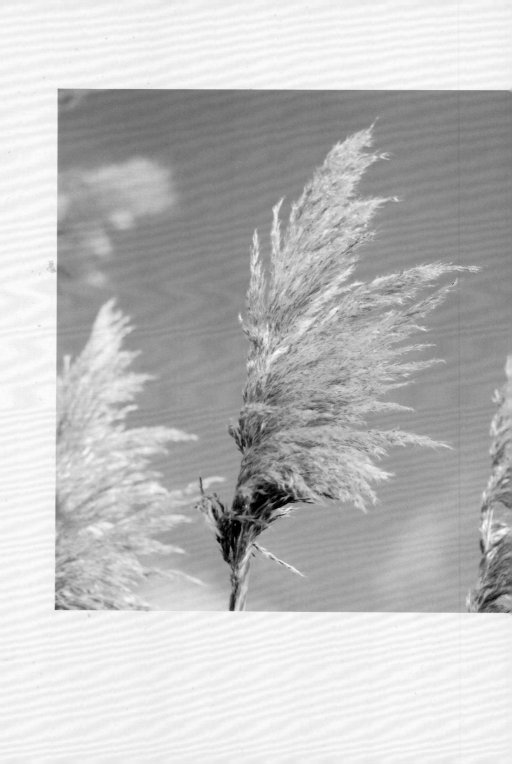

Introduction

My name is Richie Norton, and my aim is to change your life . . . or at least make it a little more magic, one little ritual at a time. Using the simple tips in this book, you can take control, reset your body, clear your mind, create new habits – and maybe transform your whole life.

Today, we have more information than ever about how to live healthier, longer lives. The secrets are out there, buried in scientific journals and research papers. But with life also being busier than ever, most people don't have the time or inclination to read them.

I wanted to put together a book that would give you scientifically proven ways to live your best and healthiest life, with the information distilled into tiny bite-sized chunks. The rituals in this book will take as little as one minute of your time to shift your habits, spark your curiosity or get you back on track. They are designed to work on both your body and your mind to produce quantifiable benefits: a healthy functional body, learning how to adapt to stressful situations, a clearer headspace, more energy, better sleep, and a more fulfilled and happier life.

But here's the magic. Once you turn these cool little health hacks into achievable daily habits and do them consistently, you can create new pathways in the brain. Over time, these neural pathways become easier to access and more instinctive. Think about cutting a path through a field of long grass or brambles. After a few cuts, the going gets easier and soon the path becomes well trodden. It's the same with behaviours. Before you know it, you will have effectively rewired your brain so the healthier habits become automatic and feel natural, and you can begin to live your life at an optimal level.

The tools in this book were born from the lessons I learned while turning my own life around. Some of you may already know me from social media or through my workshops around the world – but for those who don't, I am a former semi-professional rugby player whose dream of having a long career in the sport ended in my twenties, when I should have been in my prime. As a young guy, I took some wrong turns, lost my way and neglected my health,

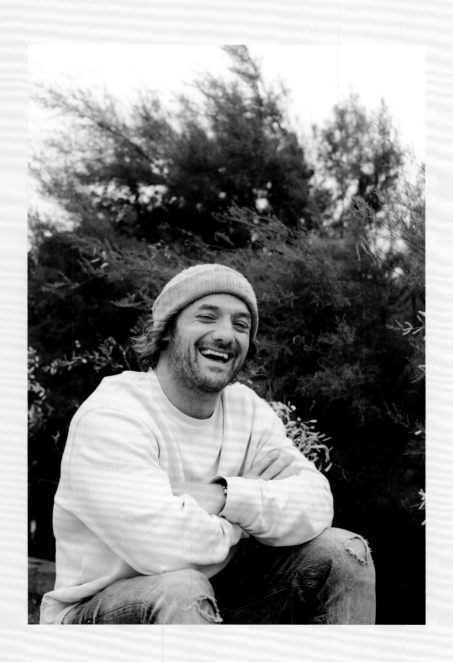

resulting in an injury that my doctors warned me would disrupt the rest of my life and meant I'd not be able to play rugby again. This broke me.

Rugby was such a big part of my life. It was more than just competing, it was my lifeline and where I felt my future was. I was fortunate to have a very active childhood, growing up in the Middle East with trips back to Europe. I remember as a kid watching my dad play rugby in the desert, and I loved getting involved in anything that involved some sort of challenge or competition. When we moved back to the UK, athletics and rugby took over my life. I loved the battles, the team bonds and the sense of purpose sport gave me. When all of this was taken away after my injury, I completely lost my way. I put on weight, drank too much, struggled to sleep and often experienced crippling anxiety that completely shut me down.

After a major health scare and a big wake-up call, I moved to Australia and made a fresh start. It was there that I discovered the things that were to save my life: surfing, yoga and the power of breathwork. Never, ever as a rugby player would I have expected to join a yoga class and enjoy it, but there I was. I was given another chance at life, found my place and was able to turn things around.

Fast-forward a few years. I'm now a human performance coach, yoga instructor and breathwork practitioner, and I get to teach all around the world sharing my story and practices. I work with sports teams, entrepreneurs and many other incredible clients, helping them optimize every aspect of their physical and mental health.

It's fair to say my life has taken some twists and turns, and it's during this wild ride that I came to understand how to look after my mind and body. I have refined and simplified the lessons I've learned along the way, and created a toolbox of uplifting rituals that you can build into your day to create new, healthier habits, even when life is hectic. These cool little vibe-heightening rituals are all backed by the latest science, and I've grouped them into one-minute, five-minute, fifteen-minute, thirty-minute and one-hour (and more) chunks, so no matter how busy life is, you can always find a way to fit something in. For example, in the time it takes you to read this page, you could do my one-minute triangle breath practice (p. 32).

Who hasn't got just one minute to prioritize their health? We only get one body to live in (as far as I know, anyway) and we're living increasingly longer. That makes it super-important to look after the precious temple that is your body, whether you're playing sport at the highest level or are more of a desk ninja that simply wants to stay sharp.

Sometimes it can feel like an overwhelming task to make the changes to your life that you want and need. That's why I wanted to make doing so as simple and quick as possible. By creating an opportunity to tick off little wins each day, you can make small, consistent steps in the right direction, and unlock a whole new level of performance. No matter who you are, and whatever your age or current level of fitness and health, you will be able to find powerful transformative ideas in this book.

This book can be a resource for life, but the first step is starting the journey, putting it all into practice, keeping it simple and getting stuck in. The changes are in four main areas: breathing, movement, nutrition and sleep. These are the four basic foundations for a healthier, more fulfilling life, and once you have these nailed, you're well on your way. Now, let's lift your vibe . . .

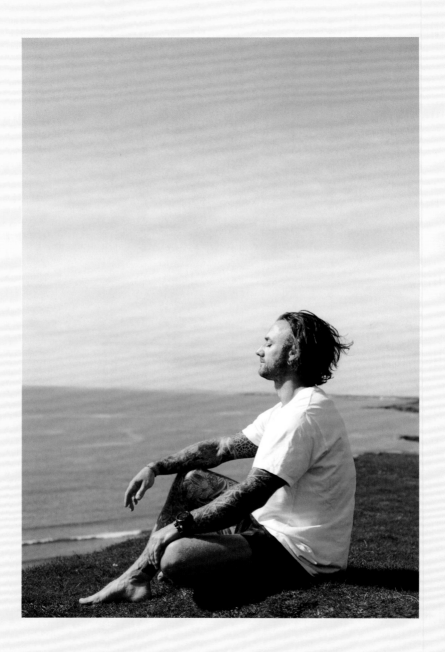

Breathing

We take around 20,000 breaths every day of our lives, but for many of us it's just another automatic process, something we never really think about. Yet most people are going through life with a dysfunctional breathing pattern that's having a huge effect on the way they feel, move, sleep and perform.

It was the same for me. During my rugby career, I was relying on skill, pure brute force, strength, and my mindset on the day. I knew very little about breathing biomechanics and biochemistry, but now realize it was my breathing dysfunction and poor breathing patterns that were a huge part of why I ran out of gas on the pitch and let a lot of potential go to waste.

A few small adjustments can massively improve the way you breathe. Taking deep, slow and controlled breaths from your belly (using your primary breathing muscle, the diaphragm), rather than short, shallow breaths into your upper chest, is a game-changer – both for your physical health and performance and your mental agility.

Breathwork practices have been around for thousands of years, but it's only now, thanks to new technology and research, that we are able to prove how powerful these practices really are.

Doing regular breathwork exercises can:
- **Reduce stress,** because it stimulates the part of your nervous system that relaxes you and calms you down.
- **Lower your blood pressure** and heart rate.
- **Reduce sensitivity** to negative emotions and anger.
- **Improve your memory** and brain function. A recent study suggested that breathing through the nose activates the part of your brain that encodes memories.
- **Help you sleep** and improve the restorative process in deep relaxation.
- **Relieve pain.**

- **Improve your skin** and boost cell regeneration by getting more oxygen around the body.
- **Give you more energy,** focus and motor control, and improve your overall athletic performance.

Breathing is now a key focus in every single activity I do, whether that's yoga, hiking, riding my bike, running, surfing, snowboarding or even working on my laptop. The more connected I am to each inhale and exhale, the more my body is in tune with what I'm asking of it – giving me the extra edge I need in order to adapt, and improving my ability to deal with those demands.

You can use breathing to find laser focus before a meeting, to calm nerves before a daunting task, to inspire creative flow, or to de-stress, wind down and get better sleep.

So why not commit to practising to improve your breath every day?

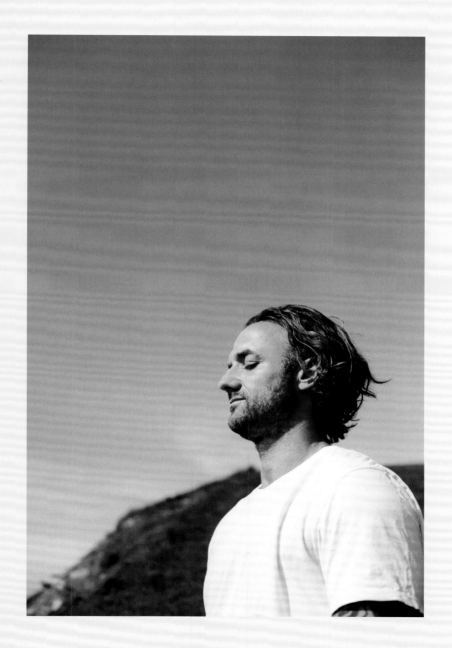

Movement

Back when I spent most weeks competing, for someone classed as a 'high performance athlete' I had surprisingly little mobility. I couldn't even touch my toes or get my arms over my head without hunching my back. Training involved throwing weights around the gym and practising on the pitch or the track.

That approach eventually led to little injuries that became bigger problems, and which ultimately ended my career. My body had no opportunity to heal and so injuries plagued me – sciatica and back pain, hyperextension of the knee, hip pain, ankle-rolling. I had poor posture and a terrible range of motion, and my body had quite simply broken from the relentless, repetitive stress I put on it.

Several years after my rugby career ended, I walked into a yoga class. That first day I struggled to do even quite basic moves. Frankly, it was embarrassing. Here I was, a 'sportsman' who looked the part aesthetically and had muscles in all the right places, but I wasn't able to move functionally or freely without pain.

I was determined to improve my mobility and repair my body, so I decided to practise those basic moves for just a couple of minutes every other day. After a few practice sessions, I noticed my flexibility improving. Within a few weeks I could keep up in the yoga class.

That was a real eye-opener for me, because it made me realize that just a few minutes of regular practice could make a world of difference to my mobility and posture. I soon noticed I was standing taller and my chest was more open, all because I'd done a tiny bit of work on my spine, hips and shoulders.

This is the message I want to pass on: it doesn't take hours of work and dedication, just consistent short practices. If you can do a short mobilization exercise first thing in the morning and another last thing at night, you will notice a huge difference to your ability to move freely. There are also big knock-on effects in other areas of life. All that extra oxygen and blood flowing around your body and to your brain gives you more energy, more headspace and more focus.

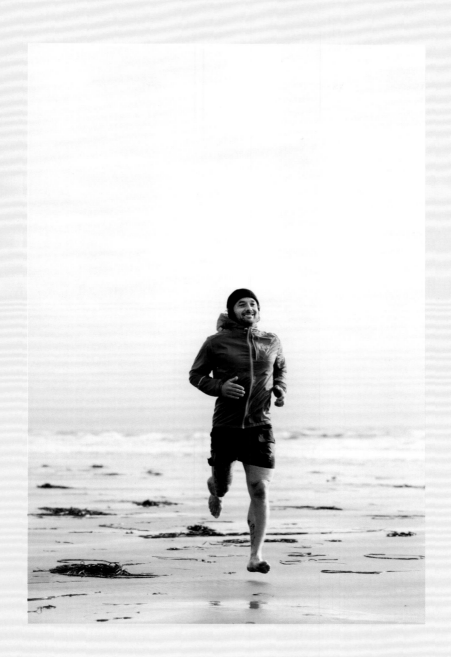

A little aside: there's a feeling sometimes that mindful exercises like mobilization, yoga, Pilates and breathwork are essentially for women in Lycra and not for your average macho rugby bloke. Thankfully, more men are getting the message that it's vital for them too, but I'd love for even more of us to step up and own this space.

We are learning more all the time about our mind–body connection, but for me, movement and mobilization has always been medicine for both the body and the mind. It's really important to move at some point every single day. So choose one of the mobilization flows from this book to do in the morning and one in the evening, depending on how much time you have, and start feeling the benefits. (You'll find five-minute versions on p. 84, and fifteen-minute versions on pp. 127 and 146.) During the day, you can keep your mobility topped up by doing a few of my 'a minute on the mat' flows (see p. 38). One minute – that's all!

Nutrition

I am not a trained nutritionist. But I have done extensive research and experimentation with my own diet over the past few years, putting my findings to the test by working closely with athletes and private clients. I have now worked out what balance of food groups and nutrients fuels my body best and sets me up for my healthiest life.

This wasn't always the case. After my rugby days I put on a lot of weight; I was still eating the big, protein-rich, carb-heavy diet that I thought I needed to build up my body, and as soon as I stopped being so active the pounds piled on. There were far too many pies, too much alcohol, too many processed low-quality meats and greasy, oily, fatty foods.

Looking back, I was overeating mindlessly most days and had no idea about portion control. And it wasn't just my weight that was affected, because the food we put into our mouths has a direct effect on our mood, our skin and hair, our sleep patterns and our energy and stress levels. All those aspects of my life were suffering.

For someone who was technically an elite athlete, I was in a sorry way. After my health scare I had a big wake-up call, and I finally found the motivation to change my diet: I cut out processed foods, I radically cut back on alcohol, I upped my vegetable intake and got smarter about nutrients. I also reduced my meat intake by about 50 per cent.

Since then, I have experimented with plant-based diets during times of intense training and also less physically demanding times. I am not vegan or vegetarian, but what I have noticed is that I have been able to cut back hugely on animal protein. I now eat predominantly plant-based proteins and I find that that approach works well for my body. It may not be exactly the same for everyone, but the latest science does tell us that those with a low-meat, majority-plant-based diet are at lower risk for heart disease, type 2 diabetes, obesity and some cancers.

I am certainly in the best shape of my life so far. And it's why the recipes I will share with you in this book are all plant-based.

Over the past couple of years, I have also experimented with other aspects of my diet after studying the scientific literature. For example, I now try to eat all my food in an eight-hour window. So on a typical day, I train first thing in the morning, then eat breakfast at around 10 a.m. I usually eat my last meal of the day by 6 p.m., making sure I had enough calories in that eating window to suit my needs. After that, my body has a break for sixteen hours until the following morning's breakfast. I have found that's enough time to give my digestive system a proper rest, which has improved my gut health and has also revolutionized my sleep because I'm not full of food late at night.

Why not look at your own eating patterns to see where you can make some adjustments? Your body won't necessarily need exactly what mine does, because no two people are identical. But if you suffer from gut problems, stress, low energy or sleep issues, or you're just not happy with your weight, maybe that's the motivation you need to make some necessary changes. It's also about understanding how you respond to certain foods, being more mindful of what you put in your body, and listening when your body says it's full.

I hope you feel inspired to try out the easy and life-changing recipes in this book. They are carefully chosen to be full of nutritious love, bursting with fibre and flavour and packed with colour in order to maximize the nutrients and turbocharge your health. Just like the rest of the book, there is something for everyone no matter how much time you have: my Midday Munch for the Mind (see p. 173) is a ten-minute winner, and my Veggie Combo Coconut Curry (see p. 209) takes less than half an hour to make.

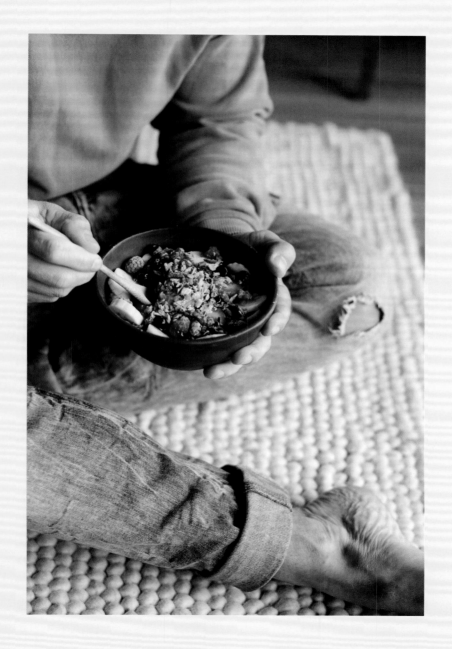

Sleep

Now it's no shock that a good night's sleep can be transformational, but how many of us are getting that precious, deep, restorative sleep? After a few years of 'burning the candle' and thinking I'd be fine running on minimal sleep, I eventually got my 'wake-up' call (pun intended) when my body shut down; I ran myself into the ground and felt like I was constantly sick with something. I'd never really respected the importance of quality sleep until I was forced to do something about it.

I was fortunate to start on the right track – I got hold of some incredible books, and managed to track down a few of the experts who are out there doing some amazing research on the subject. After going into my own sleep lab for a few months to do some experimenting, I soon realized I'd found a big piece of the 'healthy and happy life' puzzle.

Most of you know sleep is important, but did you know it's basically the key to all your superhuman powers? Yes, there will be some of you who work unsociable hours, or have young families that like to wake you up in the middle of the night, and there are also 'night owls' and others who simply don't have a choice about their sleep being adversely affected. But are you doing everything you can to maximize recovery and improve the quality of your restorative rest?

These are just some of the ways that sleep is good for our health, from the NHS:

- **Keeps your immune** system strong to fight off viruses and infections.
- **Speeds up** the healing process.
- **Reduces stress** levels and boosts mental well-being.
- **Lowers your risk** of heart disease, diabetes and high blood pressure.
- **Helps you maintain** a healthy weight.
- **Improves your** attention and concentration.
- **Increases** fertility.
- **Improves your** memory and brain function.

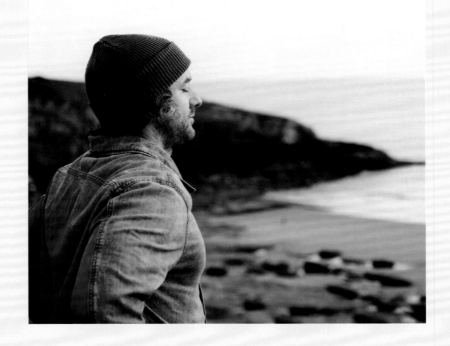

———————————— Lift Your Vibe

How to use this book

Feel free to dive in and see what catches your attention; your body knows what it needs for optimum performance, so wherever you feel drawn to is likely a great place to start.

But for those of you who like a bit more structure, my advice would be to begin with breathing. Start with the easy one-minute breath observations and go from there, as just like any other body part the respiratory system needs to be trained to be efficient – and this is the ideal base to allow you to embrace change.

You'll also want to build in some movement. How about aiming to do my five-minute wake-up flow (see p. 84) first thing in the morning and the wind-down flow (see p. 92) last thing at night? You can build up from there as your body begins to feel the benefits.

As you explore the book, you will find dozens of great ways to feel your best self – from exploring nature to mindful journaling, from cold-water therapy to a life audit, and from eating healthily to the power of connecting with friends and your community.

Keep it simple, and find the daily practices you enjoy and which best fit into your day. The book is divided up based on timing, so you can choose activities depending on whether you have one, five, fifteen, thirty, sixty minutes or more to spare. That way, there's always a little something you can do to keep motivated, and they will become new habits that stick.

I'm buzzing that so many of you want to join me on this journey, and I'm super-grateful you've taken the time to check out this book. I hope you enjoy the ride.

One-minute rituals

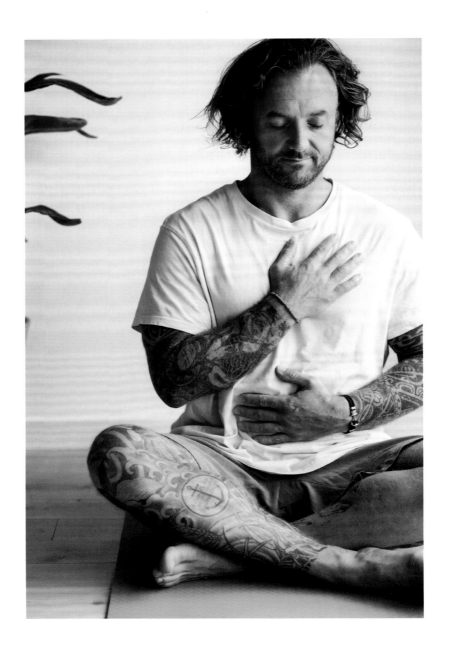

One-minute breathing practices

Our breath is a tool we can all use to improve our health. It takes some practice, so hang in there and enjoy the journey. Start with the first one-minute breath observation below, then move on to the others when it feels right. You can do these simple exercises any time: when you're waiting for the kettle to boil, or when you're standing in a queue or sitting on the bus. Set your phone alarm for a minute, but keep it out of sight so you don't get distracted. Or just keep going for as long as feels comfortable.

Breath observation

Simply observe your breath, checking in with yourself and feeling the air flowing in and out, nice and steady and controlled. Try to breathe in and out through the nose, but if you feel the need to use your mouth sometimes, that's fine. As you get more practised you'll find nasal breathing comes easier. If your mind wanders off, simply bring it back to the breath. No judgement here. Notice the slight pause between the inhale and the exhale.

The three-part breath

Here you're calling attention to the three stages of your breath, feeling it affect different parts of your upper body, one after another.

First, inhale with a steady deep breath into the lower lungs. Put your hands on each side of your belly, high enough to have your fingers wrapped around your lower ribs, and feel it expand. That's the first part of the breath. Then feel your ribs expand (the second part), and finally feel how your chest rises in the last part of that inhale. Pause briefly then exhale, reversing the process: first chest, then ribs, then belly. Pause briefly again, and repeat the cycle.

Counting breaths

The aim here is to count the length of the inhale and the exhale. Bringing your attention to the count will prevent your mind from wandering off.

Take a deep, steady breath in through the nose. Count to three as you inhale, allowing the breath to go deep into your lower lungs and feeling the expansion of the belly (put your palm on your stomach if you need to).

Now exhale, again counting to three, and feel the contraction as the air leaves your body.

The key is not to force it; it should be a smooth and steady breath in and out. If three seconds isn't working for you, choose another count that does. If you do find your mind is wandering or you feel any struggle, try breathing out through the mouth, and come back to nasal breathing next time you practise.

Triangle breaths

We're adding a pause to the breathing cycle here, so there are three corners to the breath.

Inhale for a count of three, pause and hold for a count of three, then exhale for three. Repeat that for one minute (or as many times as you like), aiming for a nice, smooth, steady breath.

As you do it, pay attention to the count and to the pause. This allows your mind to centre, to find some focus and calm. After a few practices, you might move on to counting for four seconds, then five.

I should add here that you shouldn't do breath-holds if you're pregnant, or if you suffer from anxiety attacks, as they can be triggering. Build up gradually, or just stick to the other three breathing exercises above.

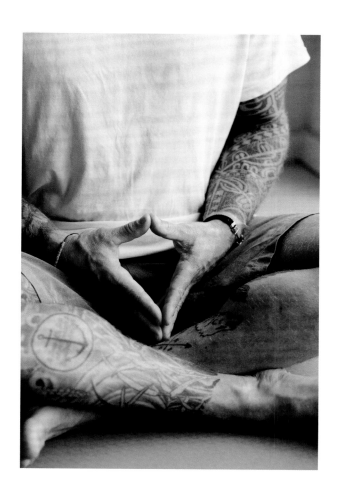

The basics of breathing

What is 'good' breathing? Here's how it looks in practice:

- **Inhale through the nose** (see below for why this is important). Not a shallow, short breath – as most will find is the norm – but deeper.
- **Feel the breath down in your belly,** not just in your chest. Your belly and ribs should expand laterally as your diaphragm (the muscle above your stomach) moves down to give your lungs room to fill with air. You should feel the pull of oxygenated air down into your lower lungs.
- **Exhale steadily,** again through the nose. Really feel the air leaving your body.

Why we should breathe through the nose

Breathing is what our noses were created to do. But it's amazing how many people use their mouths. Sometimes that's because they are unhealthy or stressed, so they get into the habit of using their mouths to pull in as much air as possible.

Or, like me, maybe they have been told that breathing out through the mouth during sport and physical exertion is 'the way of the warrior'. I certainly trained this way for many years without questioning it.

But research by some incredible breathwork experts around the world is now discovering that it's important to breathe through your nose – even during sport.

There are many reasons why:

- **Your nose warms and moistens the air,** which helps to increase oxygen flow to the lungs.
- **Your nasal sinuses produce an amazing gas** called nitric oxide. This dilates the blood vessels and allows more oxygen into your lungs and into your whole body. It can also lower your blood pressure.
- **The tiny hairs in your nose** act as a natural filter for pollutants.
- **Nasal breathing activates** the part of your nervous system that supports calm and recovery. So if you can nose-breathe even when you're exercising, you'll see some real wins. Practise first on the warm-ups and cool-downs.

Learning to nose-breathe has been a game-changer for me. It allows you to take fuller, deeper, more nourishing breaths, which helps the lower lungs to distribute more oxygen around the body. So why not try it?

If you'd like to know more about the new science of breathing, take a look at the Further reading and resources section at the back of this book.

"

———

What are you forcing in life that really isn't
right? What are you giving your time to
that you really don't enjoy? Who are you
spending time with that you know makes
you feel low? What are you putting off
because you're scared, but really you know
that it's what you'd love to do?

Answer these questions and take your first
true steps towards a happier you.

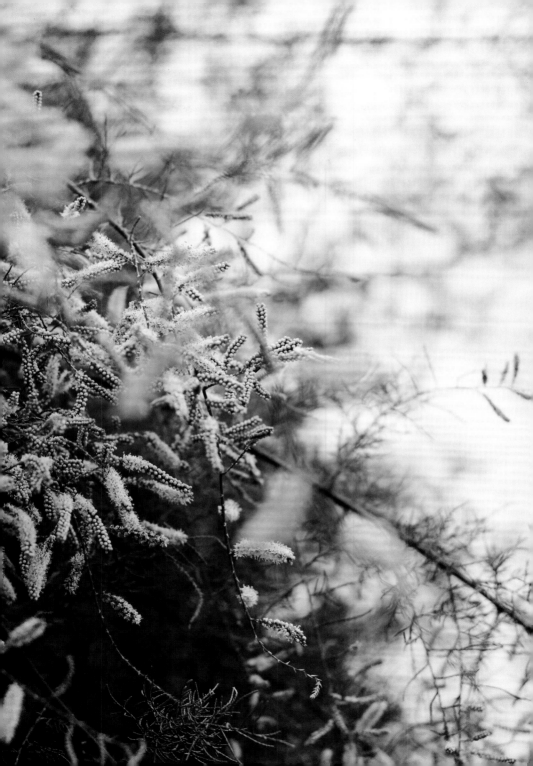

A minute on the mat

When I'm sitting at my desk working or watching TV, I'll aim to get up every twenty-five minutes and do a minute on the mat. One minute of free flow movement – that's all. I might focus that minute on my hips, spine, neck or upper body, depending on how my body is feeling and which parts feel snagged or stiff.

That micro workout completely changes the next twenty-five minutes. It fires me up, and gets the blood and oxygen flowing around my body and to my brain, allowing me to feel more switched on and alert – especially if I've been hunched over a laptop or my phone.

Try it for yourself. Choose one or two of the following exercises to do each day – or even all four if you get really hooked. You'll be rewarded with greater flexibility and an increased range of motion in just a few weeks. I do find that one minute usually becomes at least five minutes, but just start with one and see where you go.

Are you sitting (too) comfortably?

These one-minute top-up exercises are particularly important for those of you who sit for long periods. Sitting down is disastrous for your hips, shoulders, chest and spine, which are the very areas of the body that allow you to move well.

What happens when you sit is that your shoulders round and the connective tissue in your chest shortens, so your back rounds and your back muscles are put under a lot of pressure and stress. The big gluteal muscles in your bottom weaken, and your hip flexors at the front of your hips tighten. Basically, your body shuts down – not just the muscles, but deep down at a cellular level.

Scientists think that's why people who sit for hours at a time are more at risk of high blood pressure, heart disease and stroke, even if they aren't overweight. In every sixty-minute cycle, we should spend no more than forty minutes sitting. Split the remaining twenty minutes between fifteen minutes standing and five minutes moving.

Hips

After all that sitting down we're doing these days, your hips deserve some love. If you've never done anything like this before you will probably feel quite tight but that's exactly what we're here to sort out. Just take it steady and enjoy feeling looser each time you do it.

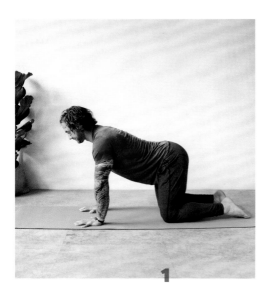

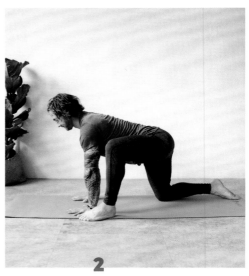

Start on all fours (shoulders above hands, hips above knees) with a nice flat back.

Bring your left foot forwards so it's flat on the ground, outside your left hand.

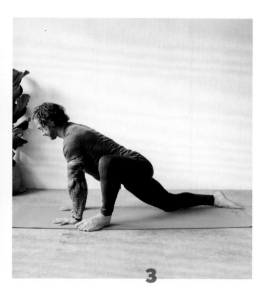

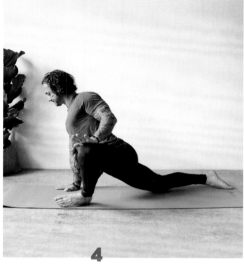

Drop your pelvis down, and notice how that pushes your upper body forwards a bit. Now gently rock your hips from side to side.

With your pelvis still dropped, put your left hand on your left knee to very gently push the knee outwards a few times. Feel your hip open a little. This is a variation of the dragon pose in yoga. Don't push it so it's uncomfortable, but apply just enough pressure to feel a stretch.

Go back to the starting position and repeat on the other side.

5

Back in your starting position, bring your left knee towards your left wrist while letting your right leg slide backwards so your hips are near the floor. Move your left foot across the body so it's more or less under your right hip. This is a variation of the pigeon pose in yoga. Lightly rock from side to side, and try to drop your left thigh and glute (the big muscle in your bottom) towards the floor.

Repeat on the right side.

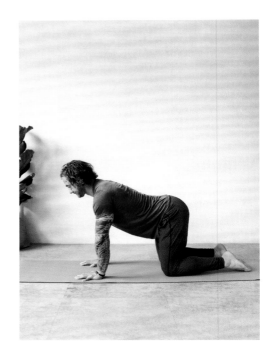

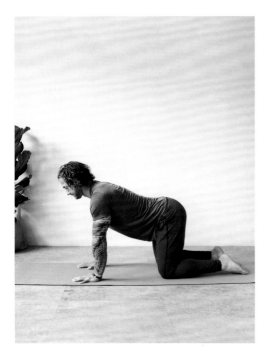

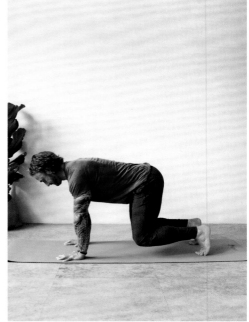

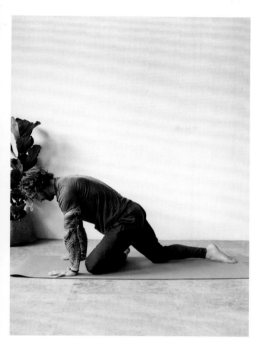

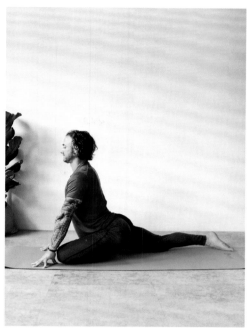

6

———

Bring your body back to all fours, then lift your knees off the ground and raise your hips into the air, heels down if possible, for one final stretch. This is the downward dog pose used in yoga and Pilates. Breathe deeply in and out while you hold this final position.

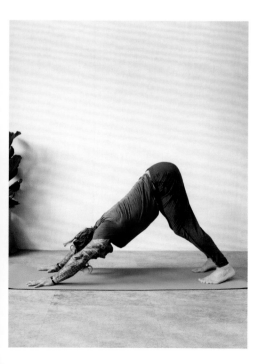

Neck

This exercise is perfect if you spend a lot of time looking at screens – which is most of us these days, right? The key here is to keep the movements slow, breathing in and out through the nose.

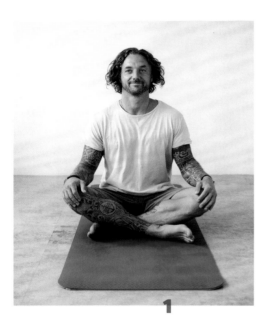

1

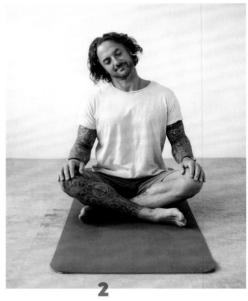

2

Sit cross-legged with your hands on your knees.

Move the head very gently and slowly to the right (feeling the stretch down the left side of the neck) then to the left. Do this a few times.

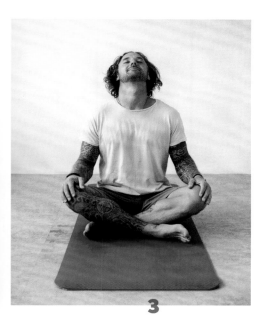

3

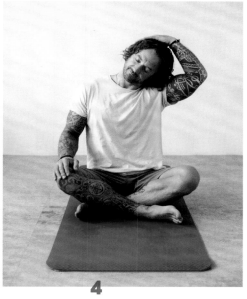

4

Stretch the neck backwards then gently forwards so your chin drops towards your chest. Repeat this, then try moving your head at different angles, diagonally forwards and backwards on the right and then the left. If there is a lot of tension in your neck, you may hear some grinding or clicking noises. Keep going, but keep it gentle.

Put your left hand over your head so your fingertips are on your right ear and gently pull down towards your left shoulder. Do the same on the other side. The key here is not to force it, but to apply a gentle pressure. As the breath moves in and out, you should feel the tension in your neck unravelling.

Repeat the moves until your minute is up.

Spine

This an essential flow for everyone, whether you spend a lot of time at a desk, looking after and juggling the kids, playing sport or putting up scaffolding. Looking after your spine is so important and can take only 1 minute!

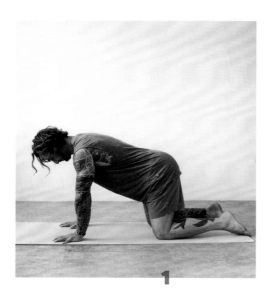

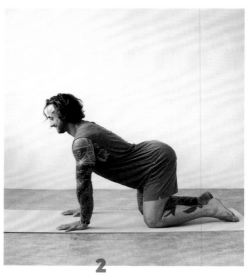

Start on all fours (shoulders above hands, hips above knees) with a nice flat back.

Breathe in as you lift your head up and tilt your hips back so your bottom sticks up.

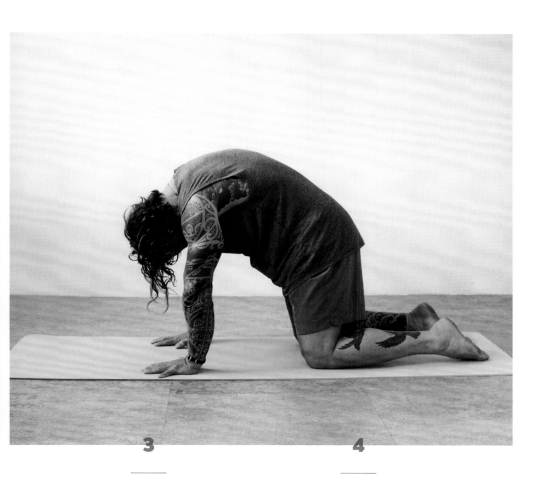

3

Now breathe out and lift your spine to the sky, tucking your chin into your chest so that your back is rounded.

4

Move between these two opposite stretches several times, really feeling the spinal articulation and gently applying a little more pressure each time. These are the cat and cow poses in yoga.

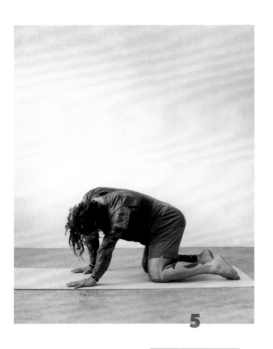

5

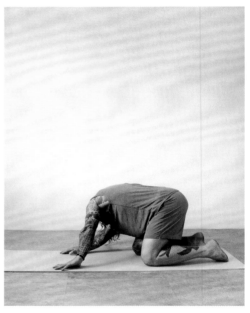

Return to all fours and add in some lateral movements
– move your hips to the right then left. Keep going,
changing the angle slightly each time, and really feel all
the different ways your spine can move. Your shoulders
and head will move too. Breathe purposefully through
the nose as you move so you control the tempo.

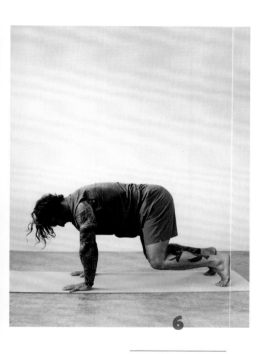

6

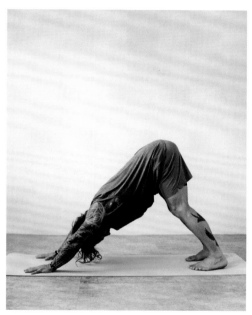

Return to all fours then lift your knees off the ground and then raise your hips up to get into downward dog. Keep your heels down if possible, and feel the stretch down your legs and back.

Repeat the moves until your minute is up.

Upper body

If you feel your shoulders are up by your ears and you're carrying tension around that area, this flow is perfect for you. Take your time leaning and releasing into each stretch to really feel the benefits.

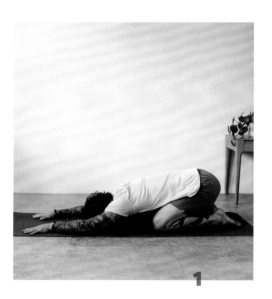
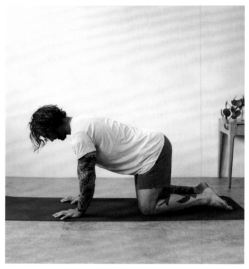

Kneel and sit back on your heels, then lean forwards so your forehead is resting on the floor and your arms are stretched out in front of you. This is a variation of the child's pose, used in yoga. Stay here for a couple of purposeful breaths, then push up to all fours.

2

Thread your right arm under your body and past your left wrist. As you reach your hand out, turn your head to the left and drop your right shoulder to the floor. This is often called threading the needle. Stay here for two deep breaths.

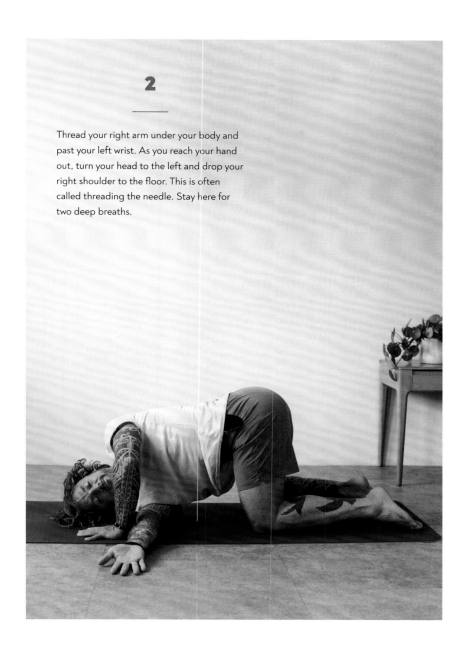

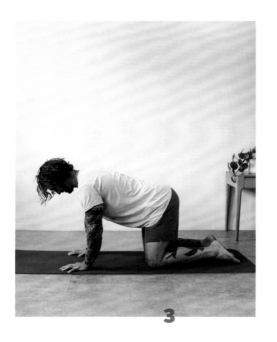

3

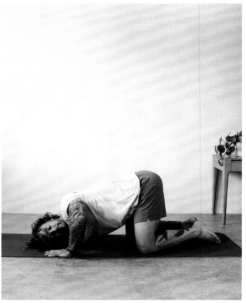

Return to all fours, then stretch your right
arm out the other way so the front of your
shoulder rests on the mat and your head is
turned to the left. Stay here for two breaths.

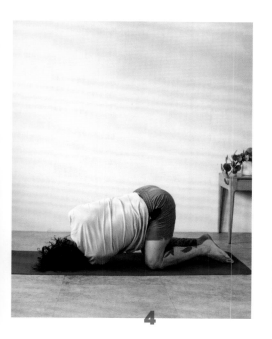

4

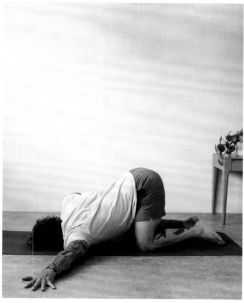

Repeat this sequence from step 2 on the other side, and don't rush it. You should feel your shoulders and upper back really opening up.

Posture fix

A must-do to iron out the tension that often builds up in your back and shoulders if you're hunched over a computer for most of the day.

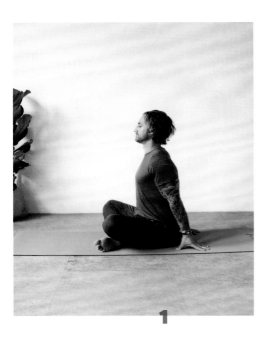

1

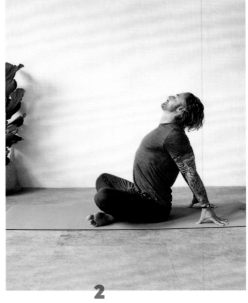

2

Sit cross-legged with your arms stretched out behind you and your hands flat on the floor. If this is uncomfortable for you, sit with your legs straight out in front of you instead.

Breathe in and push the chest forwards, and the head and neck back a little, so you feel the stretch in your chest.

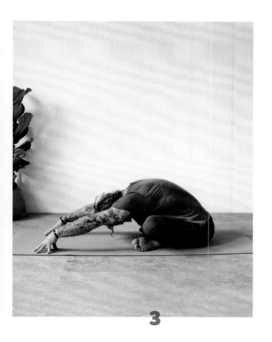

3

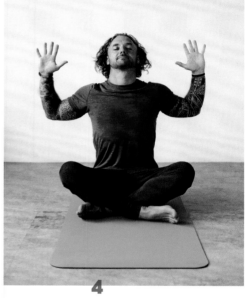

4

Breathe out and reach forwards with your arms, rounding your spine. Hold that stretch for two deep breaths.

Now breathe in and sit back up to a seated position with a straight spine, bringing your arms back so they are bent, level with your head, and your shoulder blades are squeezing together.

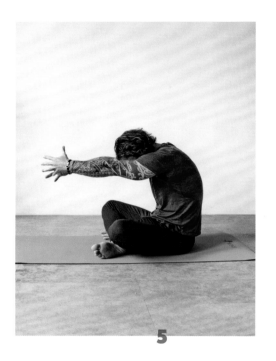

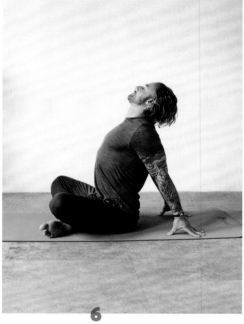

5

As you breathe out, stretch your arms
forwards again, dropping your head towards
your chest and rounding the spine.

6

Breathe in and put your arms behind you,
hands on the mat, and tilt your head back
for a long stretch, feeling the spine lengthen.

7

Then breathe out and reach forwards, arms on the floor in front of you.

Return to your starting position and do the whole cycle once or twice more. Don't rush the movements, and keep your breathing steady and purposeful.

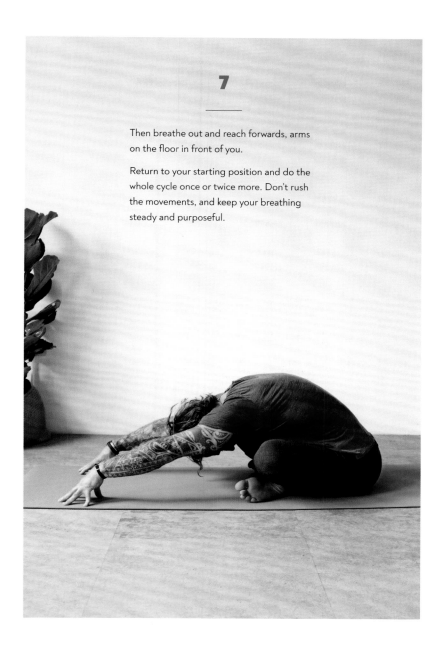

“

––––––

When asked what surprised him most
about humanity, a wise man said: 'Man.
Because he sacrifices his health to make
money. Then he sacrifices money to save
his health. He is so worried about the
future that he doesn't enjoy the present;
as a result he doesn't live in the present or
the future; he lives as if he will never die,
and then dies having never lived.'

Sometimes we need to pause for a
moment, snap out of the daily grind and
make sure we have our priorities right.

Make now count.

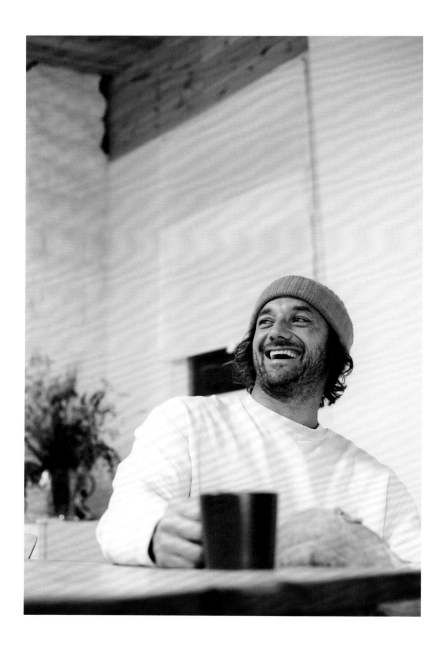

Your laughter playlist

Remember when you were a kid and you'd laugh so hard you couldn't stop? Apparently, the average four-year-old laughs 300 times a day, but by the time we're adults that's fallen to just a few times a day, if at all!

I want us all to recapture a little bit of that playful childhood joy. One way you can do this is by creating your own 'laugh list' – a collection of your favourite clips and videos from YouTube, Facebook or whichever platform you choose. Maybe you'll even include some of your own funny moments!

Find the things that really make you chuckle and lift your mood; of course, everyone's ideas on what's amusing will be different. I've recently taken to watching silly animal videos – llamas, cats, rabbits doing funny things. Ridiculous, yes. But they never fail to bring a smile to my face, lift my vibe and change my perspective, especially on a tough day when I'm in a bit of a funk.

There's some serious science behind laughter too. A genuine belly laugh is a powerful tool that can change both your mental and physical state. When you laugh, your brain releases a chemical called serotonin, known as the 'happy chemical', which lifts your mood and gives you a natural high.

Laughing also:

- **Lowers your heart rate and blood pressure,** which helps protect your heart in the long term.
- **Stimulates your respiratory system,** forcing you to take in more oxygen and deepen your breathing, which will relax and de-stress you.
- **Helps release muscle tension** that builds up during the day.
- **Cuts the levels of the stress hormones** cortisol and adrenaline in your body.

Once you've created your playlist, watch it whenever you need a little boost during the day. Or set up a daily reminder in your phone calendar. Everyone needs to laugh. No joke.

One-minute check-in

There are 1,440 minutes in a day, so aim to use just one of them to reach out to a friend. That sense of connection and community can really supercharge your life – and your health.

In one minute you could send someone a text or leave them a voice message, just saying hello and letting them know you're thinking of them. Or you could send them a photo, or a link to something you know they'd love.

It's making that connection that's important. Don't avoid friends because you feel you don't have an hour to spend on a call or a proper catch-up. It only takes a minute to reach out and reinforce the bonds of friendship. I have 'check in with a friend' on my to-do list every day, even if it just means sending them an emoji heart, smiley face or a virtual hug.

It's important to look out for each other, and it's also good for our own physical and mental well-being. Science tells us amazing things about the power of social connection.

Feeling connected can:
* **Boost your mood** and your self-esteem.
* **Lower your blood pressure** and reduce stress.
* **Strengthen** your immune system.
* **Reduce the risk** of heart disease and stroke.
* **Help you live longer.** (It's true: one key study showed that people with strong social connections were three times more likely to live longer than those with weaker connections.)

I'll take that!

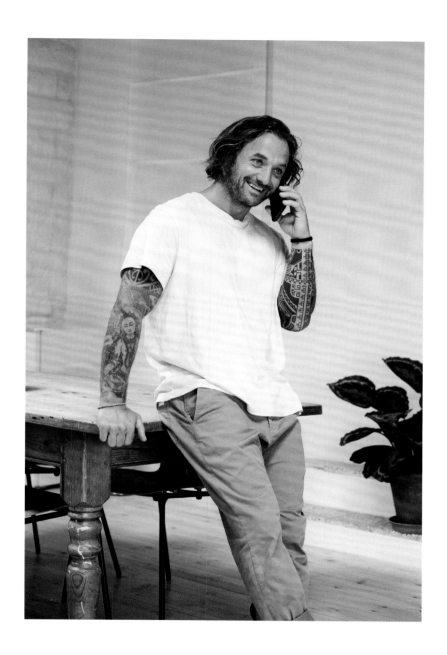

Gratitude visualization

Counting our blessings is a pretty powerful medicine for both our mental and our physical health. Research shows that practising gratitude lowers blood pressure, helps you sleep, improves your mood and reduces depressive feelings, and increases happiness and well-being. It even changes your brain for the better in the long term. Not only that, but people who show gratitude tend to eat better, take more exercise and are less likely to smoke or use alcohol.

I find a one-minute gratitude visualization when I wake up brings some calm and steadiness to my mind, especially when there's a big day ahead. I'm always grateful for my health, my family, the roof over my head, the food on my plate and the opportunity to be better than I was yesterday. We really are so lucky to be here, so putting things in perspective and appreciating what we have is so important. Don't waste a single second!

Doing another visualization last thing at night – alongside filling in my journal (see p. 108) – usually helps me sleep better too. And the effects of a gratitude practice can last for weeks! When asked to write and personally deliver a letter of gratitude to someone, volunteers in one study experienced a huge spike in happiness scores. The benefits lasted a whole month. In another, people who wrote about things they were grateful for felt more optimistic and positive about their lives. They also exercised more!

The following practices can take a while to 'feel right', but I like to think of them as life tools in my health toolbox. They're to be used when the time feels right, knowing that the more you practise them, the easier it becomes to notice the positive impact they have on your life.

Morning practice

Sit somewhere comfortable; your eyes can be open or closed. Place one hand on your chest, the other hand on your belly. Take a deep, slow, long breath in through the nose, and try to follow the progress of the air with your hands and your mind. Really try to feel the energy of the breath. Pause, then exhale – again, slowly and through the nose. Embrace the grounding feeling that comes with that steady exhalation.

Bring attention to the life-giving breath and remember how grateful you are for having the opportunity to do something great with the day ahead. Be grateful for this precious breath and feel the potential it holds – the gift that life really is.

Evening practice

'Monkey mind' is a Buddhist term for being unsettled, restless or confused. It is also the part of your brain that becomes easily distracted, so if you want to get anything done in life, you will need to shut down your monkey mind.

At the end of the day, sit on your bed comfortably and use your breath to calm that monkey mind and switch off. Place one hand on your chest, the other hand on your belly. Take a deep, slow, long breath in through the nose, feeling the air beneath your hands. Pause after the inhale, then exhale and lengthen the breath, feeling your body slowing down. Really connect to that calming, gentle breath out.

Keep following the steady breaths in and out, and know that your breath is your most precious treasure and your most incredible function. Let go of all the tension of the day, knowing that you've done your best and have no regrets. Be thankful for everything your day has brought. Tell your body it's time to rest, recover and reset. Feel grateful that you'll get another chance to live out your life in a new day tomorrow. Breathe out any feeling you need to let go of from today, and feel it drift away.

Liver cleanser

Serves 1–2

I began drinking this as a morning ritual while in Bali on my last surf trip.
The café I went to every day had it as a little shot to go with breakfast but it
was never quite enough for me, so I ended up finding out the ingredients
and making up my own batch. Now I'll do a big bottle to keep me going
for a few days.

1 small beetroot
⅓ large cucumber
2 oranges, peeled
4 large carrots
½ lemon, peeled
2.5-cm piece of ginger

Blend all the ingredients in an electric juicer. Pop a few ice
cubes into your serving glass and pour the juice over. This is a
lovely, refreshing way to start your day!

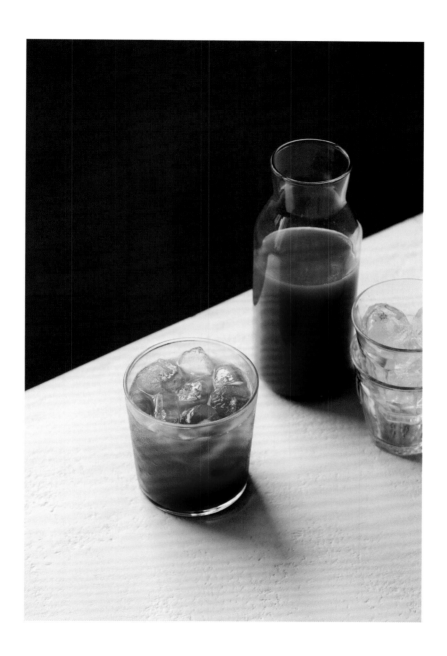

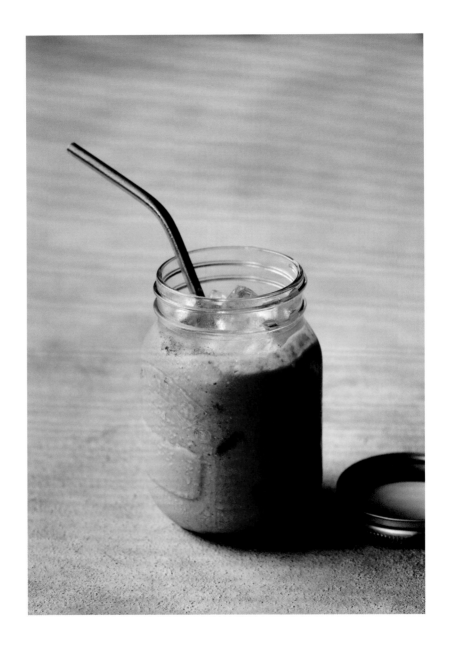

Choco-nut butter smoothie

Serves 1

The perfect way to feed my addiction to nut butter, and also give me that afternoon energy boost. This could almost be a dessert, it tastes that good. If your protein powder already contains a sweetener you might want to leave out the date to avoid it being too sweet – it's up to you!

200ml milk
2 tbsp rolled oats
1 heaped tbsp protein
    powder (20g)
1 tsp cacao (powder or nibs)
1 tsp nut butter of your choice
1 tsp chia seeds
150g frozen banana
1 medjool date, chopped
    (optional)
3–4 ice cubes

Put all the ingredients into a powerful blender and blend for at least 1 minute (or until completely smooth). Pour into your serving glass over more ice, depending on how cold you would like it, and enjoy!

Banana berry charger

Serves 2

This has evolved over the years, stemming from my gym junkie days.
I remember the original post-workout shake being loaded with protein,
and it tasted really good but this is a healthier version that you can have
any time of the day.

100g frozen banana
150g frozen mixed berries
250ml milk
2 tbsp rolled oats
1 tsp chia seeds
1 large handful baby
   spinach leaves
1 tsp honey or maple syrup
   (optional)

Put all the ingredients into a powerful blender and blend for
at least 1 minute (or until completely smooth). Pour into a
glass over ice, depending on how cold you would like it,
and enjoy!

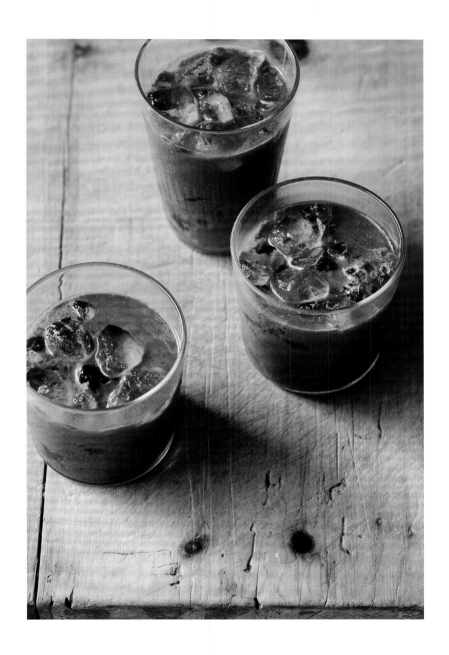

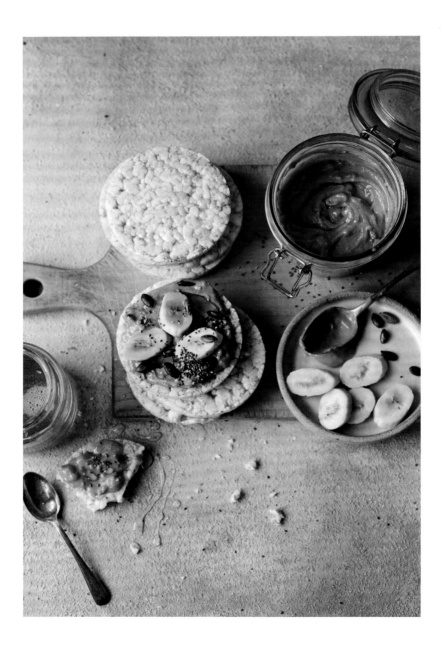

Rice cracker energy boost

SNACKS   Serves 1

A turbo snack that has saved me from my hunger attacks many times. Just the
right combination of carbs and fats to keep you fuelled-up and happy – and
ready for anything. Plus, it tastes epic!

1 wholegrain rice cake
1 heaped tsp nut butter of
    your choice
1 small banana, thickly sliced
½ tsp honey
pinch chia seeds
½ tsp toasted pumpkin seeds

Spread the nut butter all over the rice cake. Top with the
sliced banana, honey, chia and pumpkin seeds. A super-quick
energy boost, ready in just a minute.

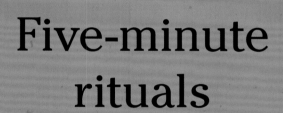

Five-minute rituals

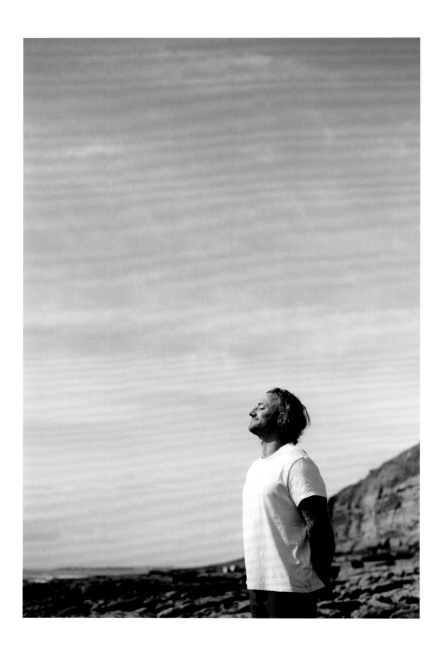

Five-minute breathing practices

Breathing should always be your first line of defence. I'd even say it could be the most powerful weapon you have to change the way you feel – whether that's to hype yourself up for the day ahead, or dial down and de-stress.

Simply spending five minutes twice a day paying attention to your breath can shift your mental state and steer you in a new, positive direction. Try it, and you'll see what I mean.

I've devised three different five-minute practices to pick from, depending on where your head is right now and where you want it to be. You can do these exercises anywhere – on your mat, at your desk, in bed, or even on your work commute (if you don't mind people staring at you!).

A few things to remember before you get started:

- **Remember to breathe** in and out through the nose.
- **If you're having trouble,** go back to basics by revisiting the introduction to breathing and the one-minute breath practices on pages 31–35.
- **If you find your mind wandering,** don't judge yourself or feel frustrated – just bring your mind back to focus on your breath.
- **It's important not to do breath-holds** if you're pregnant or suffer from anxiety attacks, or if you're finding them uncomfortable. Be intuitive, and listen to your body.

Alert and focused

This practice will help you find more focus, and bring you to an alert state. You can also use it when you wake up or as a little check-in to calm nerves before an important meeting or task. What we're doing is adding a pause at the top of the inhale and at the bottom of the exhale. This is called box breathing.

Start with a count of four: inhale for a count of four, hold for four, exhale for four, then hold again for four. Repeat this for five minutes.

When you bring a hold into a breath practice, it makes you very present. While you're starving the body of oxygen and carbon dioxide builds up, it's very hard to think of anything else and so your mind can't wander.

If a count of four feels too much, start at two or three. Choose a pace and a length of hold that suits you; it shouldn't be too much of a challenge or feel too stressful.

Reset and de-stress

Try this when you feel a little bit anxious. Maybe stress has started to build up in your body, or you're in an intensive environment and feel triggered. This five-minute practice will allow you to reset and find your 'normal' again.

Inhale and count down: 4, 3, 2, 1. Leave a short pause at the top of the inhale, then let that breath release with a steady and gentle exhale for double the count. So breathe out for 8, 7, 6, 5, 4, 3, 2, 1, then have another little pause. Repeat the cycle for the full five minutes — or as many times as you need until you feel calm.

Try your best: it may be that in each cycle you find one breath is longer or shorter than you were aiming for, but don't let that bother you. The idea is to take control of your breath – to literally 'catch' your breath – which will physically calm you down.

Wind-down

You can use this practice when you're recovering after a workout or when you're preparing for bed. What you're doing here is adding a breath-hold at the top of the inhale, and lengthening the exhale. Try to make that exhale as long and steady as possible, which will help you feel calm and present.

So, start with an inhale of 4, 3, 2, 1. Pause and hold for 4, 3, 2, 1, then gently exhale for 8, 7, 6, 5, 4, 3, 2, 1. Add a tiny pause at the bottom of that exhale as

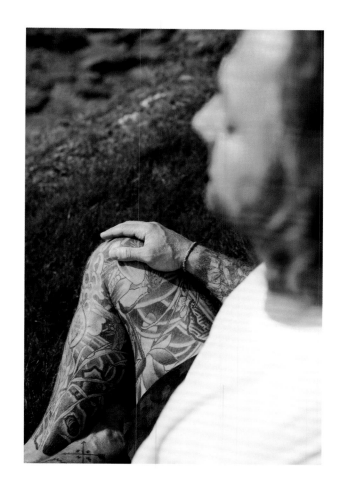

you reset, then inhale for a count of four and repeat the process.

The idea is to keep it smooth and steady as you calm the nervous system down, so it's important to find a tempo that works for you. You may find when you start out that you feel quite sensitive to the carbon dioxide build-up when holding your breath, so reduce the hold to a count of three or even two if you need to.

I don't always have a plan with my breathing exploration. It depends on where I'm at mentally, or the task at hand. But no matter what the focus or intention, paying attention to my breathing always seems to give me control over my body and my mind.

With breathing, you can begin to sense changes in your behaviour, and physical sensations become a warning signal to check yourself. You can decide to steer yourself in a new direction – you have the tools to do so – and that's a superpower.

A word about mornings

The way you treat yourself in the morning really has a powerful impact on the rest of your day. Setting a good vibe first thing can make all the difference.

I like to set my alarm for at least fifteen minutes earlier than I need to. When I get up, I rehydrate my body and brain with a large glass of water with fresh lemon juice and a pinch of Himalayan salt, then I do my 'alert and focused' five-minute breathing followed by a five-minute flow on the mat and five minutes of journaling (see p. 108). After that, I'm ready for anything the day brings, and I am able to start my day positively and intentionally.

Science tells us that, for most people, mornings are the brain's most productive time – even if you don't think they are – so it makes sense to harness those powers as efficiently as possible. Try it: you may be surprised just how powerful those extra fifteen minutes can be.

"

Some days you may need to step into some dark places and tune out the distractions. This is often when we're able to delve deeper and access a source of power that only comes from facing the uncomfortable, and from calling on past challenges we've overcome. This is when we force our body and mind to adapt, pushing through those signals to stop.

Growth comes when you push your boundaries and move past your perceived limits, and for this to be possible WE MUST LEAN IN and block out the noise.

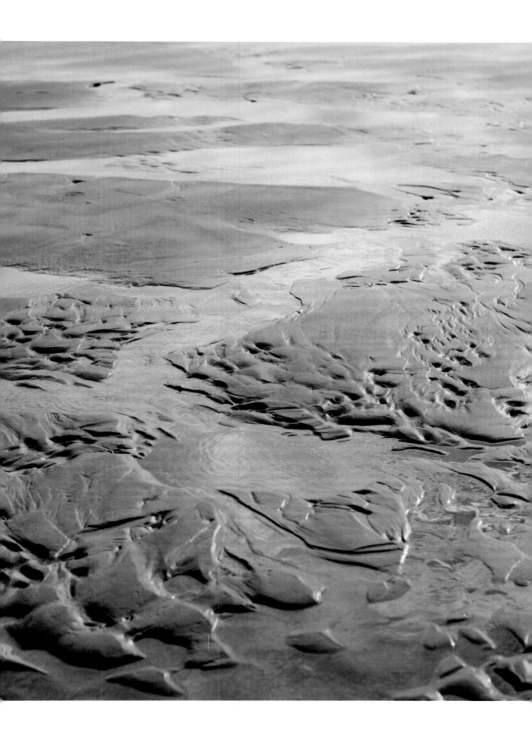

Five-minute flows

If you can spend just five minutes first thing in the morning stretching and moving, you will lubricate your joints, get blood and oxygen flowing around your body, clear your head and set yourself up for a good day.

Doing the wind-down flow (see p. 92) in the evening will 'down-regulate' your system (steady the mind, slow the heart rate and calm your vibe), allow the mind to quieten, begin to relax you, and soften tension in the body and prepare you for sleep.

Do these two flows every day for a week, and you'll notice how much better your body and mind feel. Next thing you know you'll be feeling sharper, buzzing about, and basically be an unstoppable Jedi ninja badass. Or something close.

So put on some music that puts a smile on your face, take your time and sink into each movement. Keep breathing mindfully and purposefully – always through the nose.

Don't worry about how flexible or mobile you are at the beginning. That will come. Before I discovered mobility training, I couldn't even touch my toes. (Nowhere near, in fact! Maybe just past my kneecaps on a good day . . .) But trust me – the journey is worth it.

Wake-up flow

This gentle movement practice is such a great way to start the day, getting the blood circulating from your head to your toes, lengthening and opening up your body and preparing you to take on the world and be at your best.

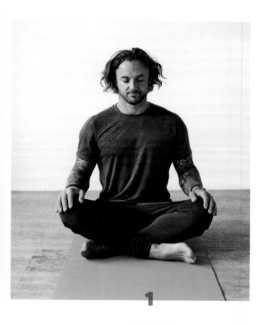

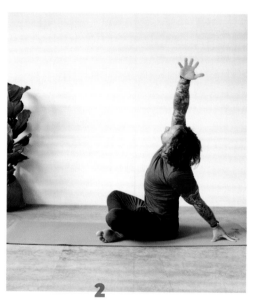

Start sitting cross-legged on the mat. Take a few deep breaths in and out through your nose, and follow each breath cycle – the steady inhale and gentle exhale.

Place your left arm out behind you, hand on the floor, and stretch your right arm over your head, feeling your right side open up. Hold that stretch for a breath, then repeat on the other side.

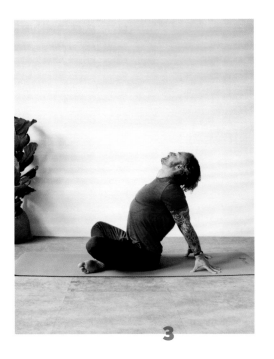

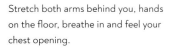

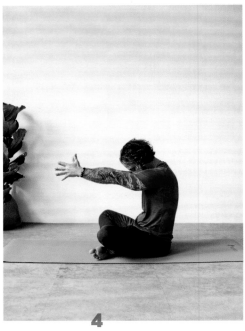

Stretch both arms behind you, hands on the floor, breathe in and feel your chest opening.

As you breathe out, drop your chin to your chest and reach forwards with your arms, pushing your back away.

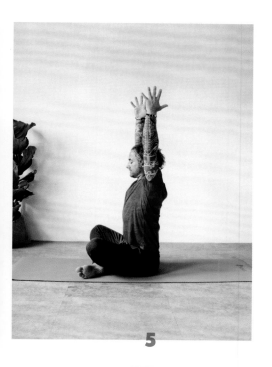

5

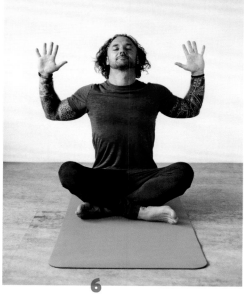

6

Inhale and put your arms straight up.

As you exhale bring your arms down with elbows bent and your hands by the side of your head (the cactus position). Inhale and open up the chest, squeezing your shoulder blades together.

Then, as you exhale, repeat from step 4 and reach forwards with your arms. Inhale and reach your arms up, then exhale back to cactus.

7

Flip onto all fours, hands under your shoulders with fingers nice and wide, knees under your hips. Take a breath in, tuck your toes under and hover your knees above the ground. As you breathe out, lift the hips high and straighten your arms (downward dog position). Try to keep your heels on the ground, then make little stepping movements with your feet, one at a time, stretching the back of the calves.

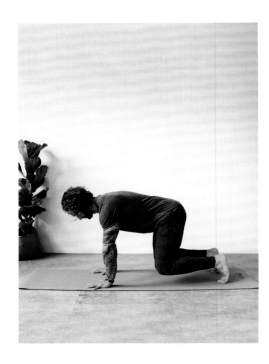

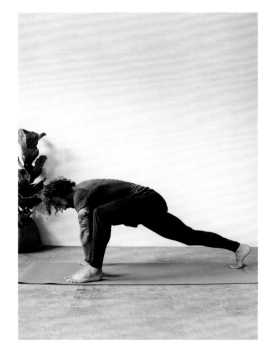

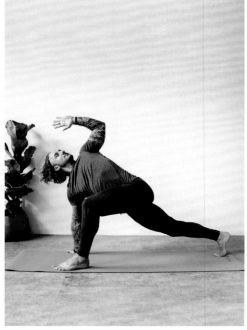

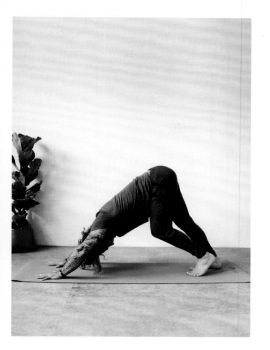

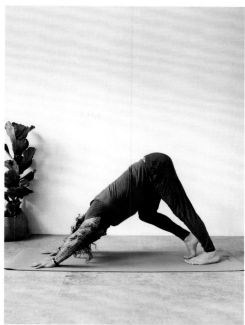

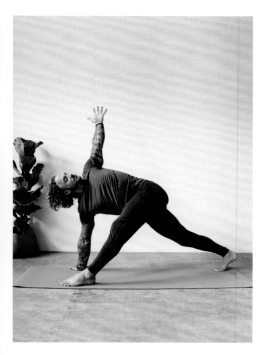

8

Take a breath in and, as you do so, step the left foot forwards so it's outside your left hand. (If you can't manage this in one smooth movement, you can use your hand to help.) Turn your right hand outwards to support you, take a breath in, and rotate your torso to the left, releasing the left arm and keeping it bent. Breathe in, and on the next breath out, straighten the left leg and extend the left arm into the air.

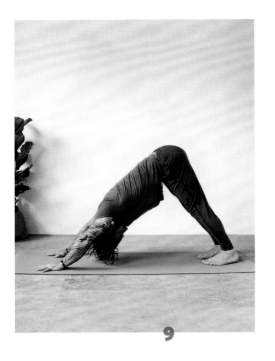

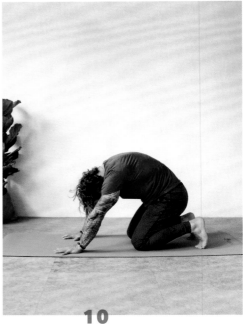

9

10

Put the left hand down again and step back with your left foot, pushing into downward dog. Keep the hips nice and high and feel the body really lengthen. Now repeat step 8 with the right foot and end in downward dog.

Go back to all fours and move your spine up and down and hips left and right, really feeling the body opening and stretching.

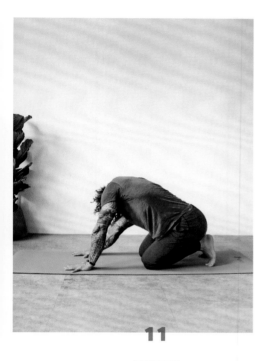

11

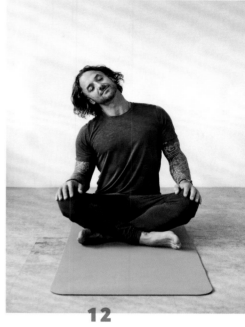

12

Let your body move freely in all directions, keeping your hands and knees on the ground.

Finish the practice by going back to your cross-legged sitting position. Put your hands on your knees and wind down by moving your head and neck, then your shoulders, gently from side to side, taking a few controlled breaths in and out.

Now you're good to go.

Wind-down flow

This will help you down-regulate and find some calm for both the mind and the body. Do it during a stressful day to bring you some chill time, or at the end of the day to help you wind down and prepare for sleep. Hold each move in this flow for two to three breaths, or up to five if you have time.

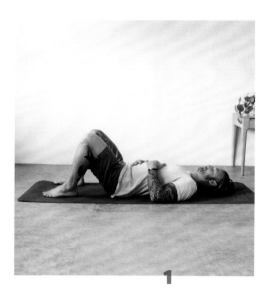

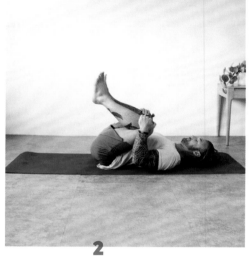

Lie down on your back, knees bent, and round your back down into the mat. Put your hands on your belly and take some deep breaths in and out through the nose. Make the out-breath longer than the in-breath with this flow to maximize relaxation.

Bring your knees up and squeeze them into your chest. Hold for a couple of breaths.

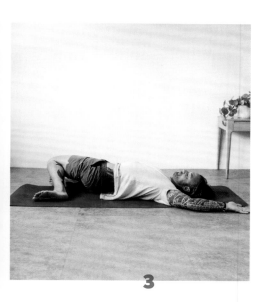

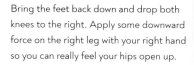

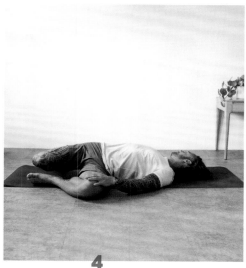

Bring the feet back down and drop both knees to the right. Apply some downward force on the right leg with your right hand so you can really feel your hips open up.

Repeat on the left, and do this two or three times more on each side.

5

Move your feet back to the floor with your knees bent. Then inhale and raise your hips off the floor, moving your arms overhead with the backs of your hands on the floor. Exhale and bring your hips back down and your arms back to your sides, palms on the mat. Repeat this twice more.

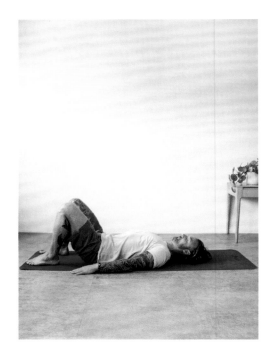

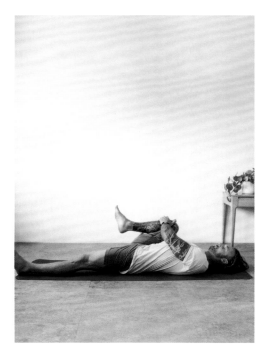

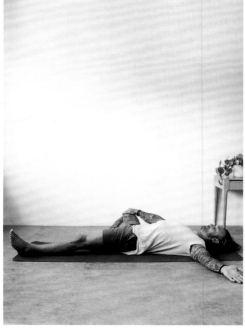

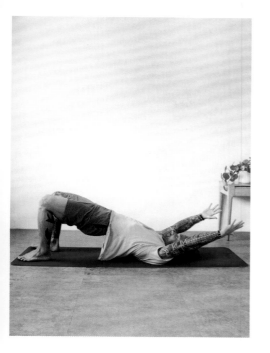

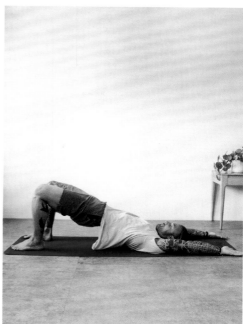

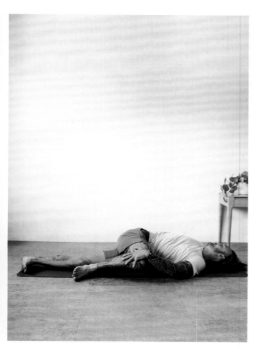

6

Bring your right knee towards your chest
and hold it with your hands while you stretch
out your left leg on the floor. (If this is too
much for your hips, keep the left leg bent
and your left foot on the floor.) Stretch your
left arm out and push your right knee out to
the side with your right hand, feeling the
space open up in your hips. Hold for a
couple of breaths, then put your left hand
on the right knee and gently pull your right
leg across your body, twisting so you get a
good stretch across the chest and back.

Repeat the sequence with the left leg.

7

Cross the right leg over the left knee (your left leg should be bent with the foot flat on the floor). Pull on the left thigh with both hands, so your left foot leaves the floor, if you want to feel an extra stretch in your right glute. Keep the pressure level so your right shin stays more or less parallel to the floor. Rock gently from left to right.

Repeat with the other leg.

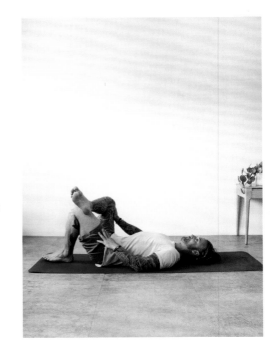

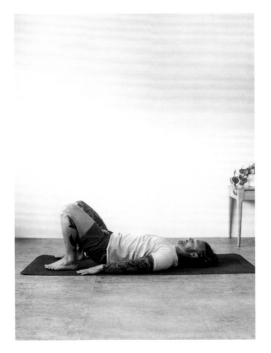

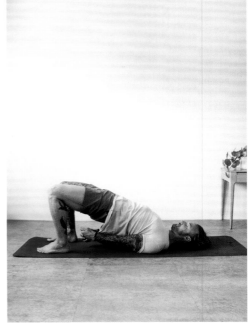

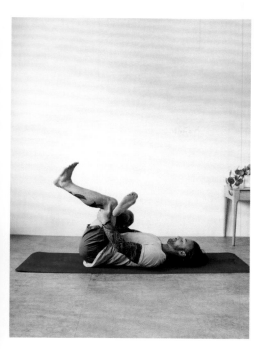

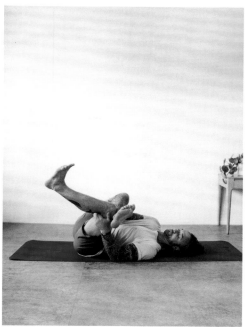

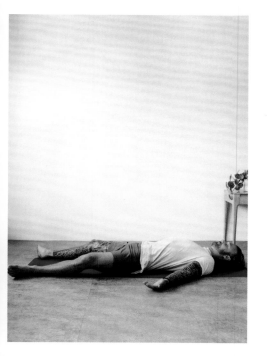

8

Return to the starting position. Inhale and raise your hips off the floor. You may need to bring your feet slightly closer to your body here. Now 'walk' up onto your shoulder blades so you're in a bridge position. Interlock your fingers under your body, bringing the elbows towards each other.

Finish by lying flat on the mat, letting your legs and arms relax and roll out. Find some stillness. Breathe steadily in and out several times, grounding yourself a little more each time.

Desk flow reset

If you're working at a desk, it's always best to get up and move around regularly. But if you can't, this flow is an effective quick fix for your posture – it will help open up your hips and back, and boost your energy by improving your circulation. Do this flow as often as you like, but aim for twice in a working day. This exercise sequence is designed for you to follow along in your chair.

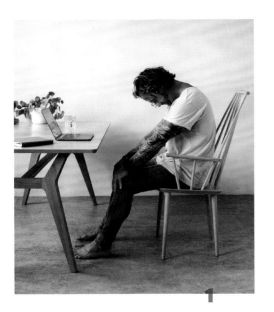 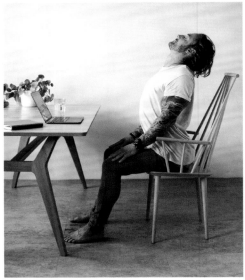

First, we're going to reverse that hunch you get from sitting down for long periods by doing some quick spinal waves. Put your hands on your knees and round your spine, then move your shoulders back and straighten the spine. Move smoothly between these two positions.

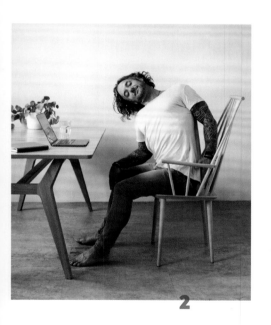

2

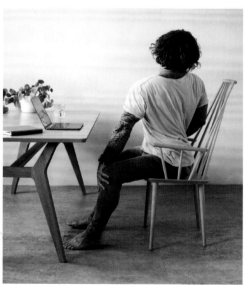

Then move each shoulder separately, upwards and outwards, leaning forwards then backwards so you really mobilize and warm up the spine. Try to create a nice, fluid spinal flow.

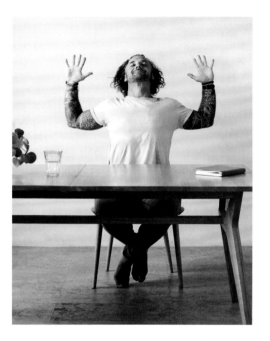
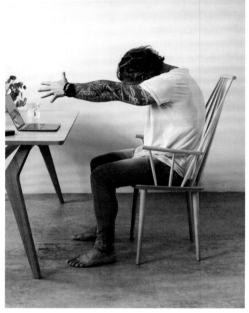

3

Inhale and pull the shoulders back. Your arms should be bent, with your hands at the side of your head (cactus position). Exhale and stretch the arms forwards. Do this four more times. Now hold the stretch as you reach forwards for a few seconds, then hold the stretch with your arms back, breathing space into your shoulders and spine.

4

Put your hands on the back of your chair
seat, near your bottom, and breathe in
deeply, feeling your chest expand and giving
the shoulders a chance to open. Exhale,
relax and then repeat twice more.

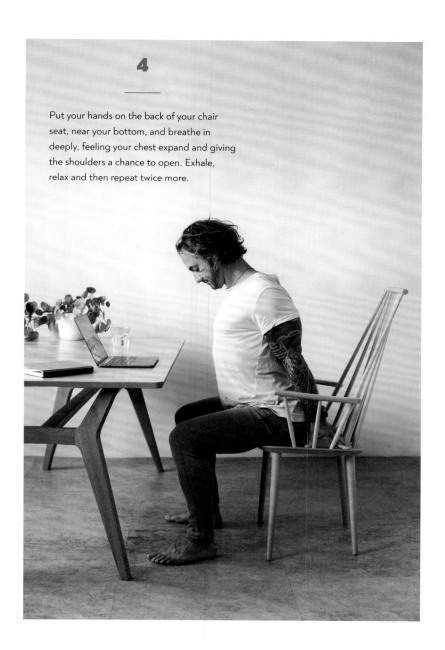

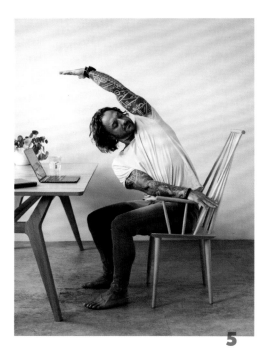
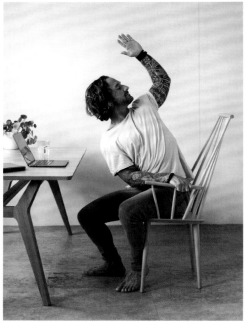

5

Move your right hand across your body and grab the left arm of your chair (if your chair hasn't got arms, hold the outside of your left thigh). Raise your left hand over your head, and feel the stretch down your left side. Hold, then inhale and pull the left arm back, bending it at the elbow and twisting your body to the left, looking over your left shoulder, if you can.

Repeat this sequence on the other side. The key is not to rush this flow; let your breathing control the tempo.

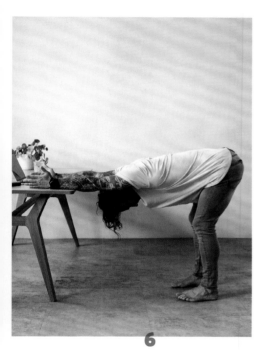

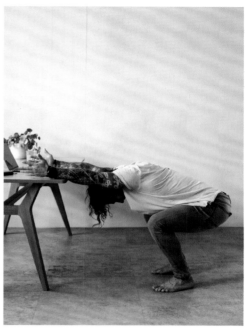

6

If you can, stand up and step away from your desk, bending at the waist and resting your arms on the desk. Bend your knees and drop slightly, then return to the starting position. Repeat two or three times.

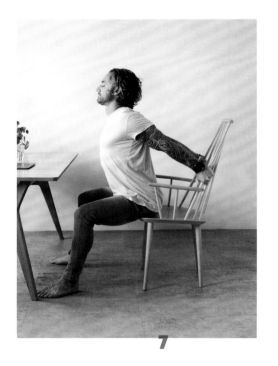
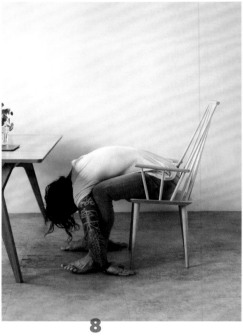

7

8

Sitting down again, open your chest and try to straighten your arms behind you, bringing your shoulder blades together and opening up the chest as you inhale. Now relax, bringing your arms forwards again and rounding your shoulders as you exhale. Repeat twice more.

Stretch forwards towards the floor to give your spine some extra decompression.

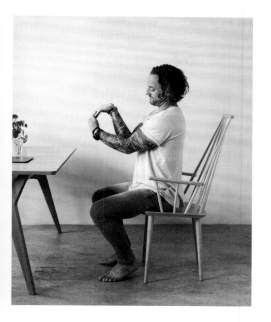

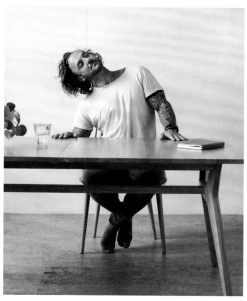

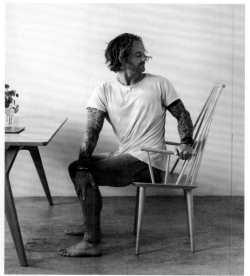

9

Give the wrists some love by twisting and rotating them.

Finish by sitting back up, rolling your shoulders a few times each way, rolling your head in a few gentle circles, and twisting your upper body from left to right.

"

―――――

A few minutes a day keeps the Zimmer frame away. We're all going to move a little differently, but we shouldn't neglect working on mobilizing and stretching – no matter where we're starting from. If you feel pain or discomfort, move around it and progress from there. Build a better connection with your body and you'll soon see and feel the rewards.

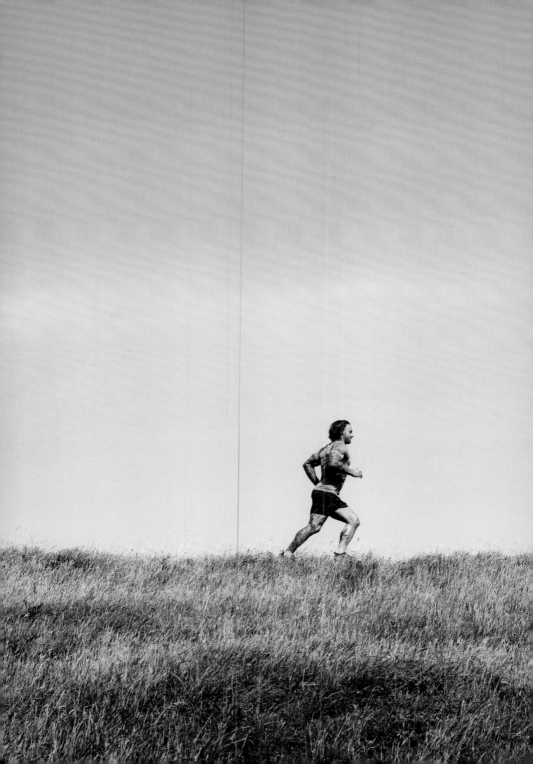

The five-minute journal

If there's one small thing that's changed my life in the past few years, it's this. For at least five minutes a day, I fill in my journal. Not tons of words, and no massive effort: just a few bullet points first thing in the morning and last thing at night, and I'm done. But the effect has been huge. I feel more focused and energized, I'm grateful for everything in my life (even on days that don't go so well) and I sleep like a baby.

It might sound a bit left-field, but research in the field of positive psychology has shown that writing a journal that has a gratitude element to it can:

- **Make you happier** and more positive.
- **Help you handle** change better.
- **Make you calmer** and less stressed.
- **Help you to sleep** better.
- **Reduce physical pain** if you're ill, and strengthen your immune system.

And here's how to do it . . .

1. **Find something to write on.** You don't need anything fancy – you can even use sticky notes if you want, although having a notebook is better because it's like creating a map of your thoughts that you can look back on in the weeks and months ahead. You can buy ready-made journals, or create your own in a notebook and use a page a day.
2. **When you wake up,** put the date at the top, then underneath write 'I am grateful for . . . ' and list three things. They might be 'my healthy body – can't wait to get it stronger', 'my warm bed' and 'the love of my mum'. Anything!
3. **Underneath, write** 'Things to make today amazing . . .' followed by another list of three. They don't have to be huge ambitions; small goals can be wins too. Maybe 'to check in on my friend Alex', 'get to bed before 10.30 p.m.' and 'buy veg from the market'.

4. **In the evening before you go to bed,** create the heading 'Great things that happened today . . .' and list three successes – however big or small. Maybe that's 'my boss praised my work', 'I felt the warm sun on my face' and 'I got out for a run'. If you've had a bad day, all you might be able to write is: 'I survived. But I did make some time to go for that walk and I did drink more water than usual and I made sure I had veggies at lunch.' Those are all wins.

5. **Underneath, write** 'How could I have made my day better?' List three things that you wish you'd done differently or handled better: for example, 'listened to my kids calmly rather than going off on one', 'got up twenty minutes earlier and made it "me time" before anyone else was up' and 'got enough sleep the night before so I felt energized'.

That's it! All it takes is five minutes a day for the magic to work.

I am grateful for . . .

_____

_____

_____

Things to make today amazing . . .

_____

_____

_____

Great things that happened today . . .

_____

_____

_____

How could I have made my day better?

_____

_____

_____

There are a couple of key points to bear in mind:

- **Write it soon after you wake up.** You've got about an hour when your mind is at its clearest and most receptive, so make the most of it. Being positive in that little window sets you up with a good mindset. You're short-circuiting negativity before you kick off your day.

- **Journal every day.** You're tired? You had a late night? You're running late? Do it anyway. Everyone can spare a couple of minutes, no matter how busy they are. Making it a habit creates positive neural pathways in your brain, and it will get easier the more you do it.

So why is morning and evening journaling so powerful?

By reaching for your pen when you wake up and writing down what you're grateful for, you're putting things in perspective and reminding yourself that life is great – even on bad days. You're building an optimistic pattern of behaviour and creating more positive energy as you start your day – so you'll be looking for better outcomes rather than dwelling on stuff that can really pull you down and leave you in a low vibration.

In the evening, you're bringing your mind back to the things that went well, even if your day hasn't been the best. By writing how you could have made things better, you're processing what's happened and making peace with the day – but you're also creating the building blocks for the next day. You can go to bed feeling calm and clear-minded and ready for sleep, rather than lying awake with too many 'mind apps' open, ruminating and stressing.

Journaling allows you to start and end your day with positivity, no matter what happened in the middle. And science shows us that positivity can lead to better physical and mental health.

All this, from five minutes' effort!

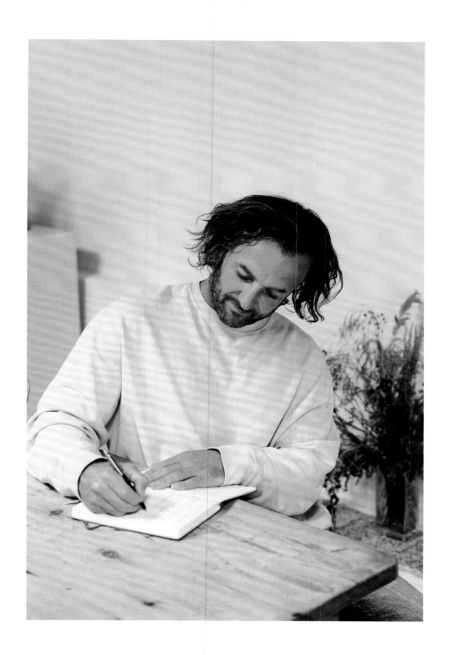

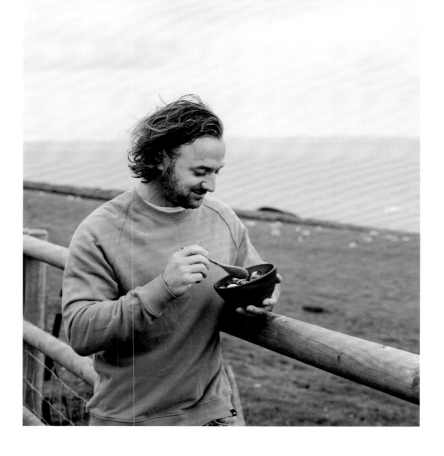

A morning nature fix

I'm a country bumpkin at heart and nature is my favourite place to hang out. It makes me feel safe, connected, at peace and completely free.

All of us need a nature fix every day, even if you live in the city and can't see green from your windows. So I want you to make a promise to get outside for just five minutes in the morning, or allocate some time in your day for a nature escape. Take your cup of tea or breakfast to the garden or balcony, or walk to any local green space – whatever access to the outside you've got – and absorb nature.

Leave your phone inside and just take in your surroundings, using all your senses to notice what's going on around you: the wind on your face, the leaves rustling in the trees, the birds moving across the sky.

Breathe deeply and steadily through your nose, and try to feel that connection with the natural world. It works like a mini meditation. If it's not too cold, you can go barefoot and feel the grass beneath your feet, 'earthing' yourself.

There's true magic at work here, and it's all backed up by science . . .

Getting natural daylight as soon as possible after you wake up stops your body producing the sleep hormone melatonin in the daytime. That will help your body clock stay in tune, and help you get better sleep that night. Sunlight also feeds your body the vitamin D it needs to stay healthy.

Being in nature does all kinds of incredible things to your body:
- **It distracts your mind** from negative thought loops.
- **It's been shown to reduce stress** hormone levels, which calms the body's fight-or-flight response, and can lower blood pressure.
- **It cuts your long-term risk** of type 2 diabetes, cardiovascular disease and premature death. You don't need a forest in your garden, either; one study found you could get the same benefits from urban green areas.

So, find what works for you and try to get outside each morning.

66

———

Train your mind like you train your body.
When the two are working together and
both are cared for in the same way . . .
magic happens. Don't put so much
pressure on yourself when beginning a new
challenge or starting your health and
fitness journey. Listen to your body and
mind, and feel what they need each day.
Know that simple daily habits can have a
huge impact on all aspects of your life.
Give it time, and learn what works for you.

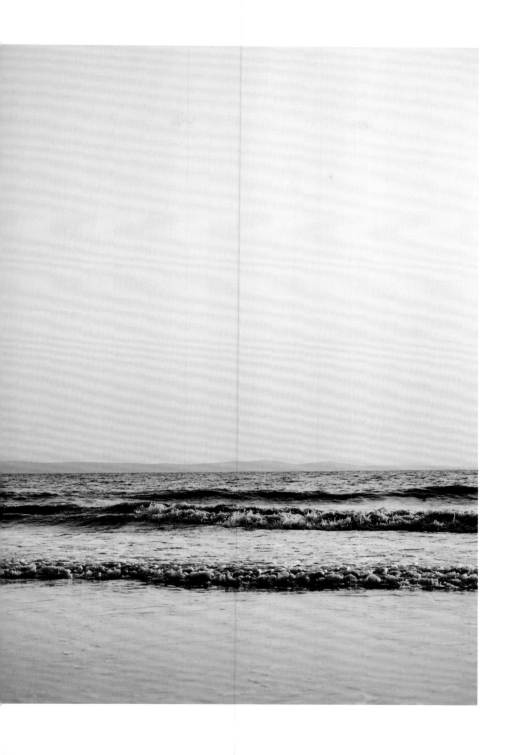

Green smoothie bowl

Serves 2

I've had a few smoothie bowls while on my travels, and it's become the best quick fix to get some nutrients in and mix up the breakfast routine. I know that eating your greens isn't for everyone, but I find this super-simple recipe is a tasty way to keep your body and mind healthy.

1 large ripe avocado
200g frozen banana
150g frozen mango
100g baby spinach
1 handful mint leaves
2 tbsp milled flaxseed
juice of 1 lime
100ml oat milk
50ml water
1 tsp spirulina powder (optional)
1 tbsp agave syrup

Toppings
1 kiwi fruit, peeled and sliced
4 strawberries, hulled and sliced
1 tbsp chia seeds
4 tbsp granola

Cut the avocado in half and remove the stone. Scoop the flesh directly into a blender. Add the banana, mango, spinach, mint and flaxseed. Pour in the lime juice, oat milk, water, spirulina (if using) and agave. Blend until smooth and then spoon into two serving bowls.

I love topping this with kiwi fruit, strawberries, chia seeds and granola, but you can use your own favourites!

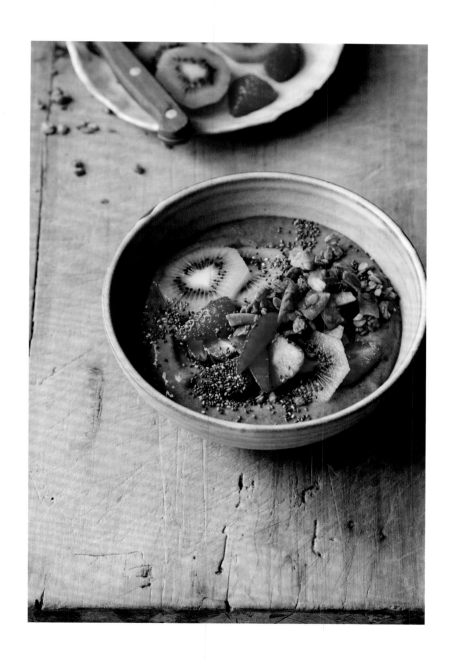

Hot chocolate treat

Serves 1

This is a fairly new love affair. Since trying chaga at a retreat a few years ago, I've delved deep into the health benefits of these medicinal mushrooms that are making a big impression on the health and well-being world: they're packed with fibre, low in calories and a natural source of antioxidants. But if you can't get hold of it this recipe is still a real treat with just cacao.

50ml boiling water
1 tsp chaga mushroom powder (optional)
2–3 tsp cacao powder (depending on whether you use chaga or not)
pinch ground cardamom
pinch ground cinnamon, plus a pinch to serve
1–2 tbsp maple syrup
150ml oat milk
50ml oat cream

Pour the boiling water, chaga (if using) and cacao into a small saucepan and mix well. Add the remaining ingredients and cook on a gentle heat. Once it's brought up to a simmer, whisk well for 1 minute to create some froth. Pour into your favourite mug, sprinkle over a pinch of cinnamon and enjoy.

Alternatively, if you have one of those electric milk frothers at home, you can just pop all the ingredients in and it will work a treat!

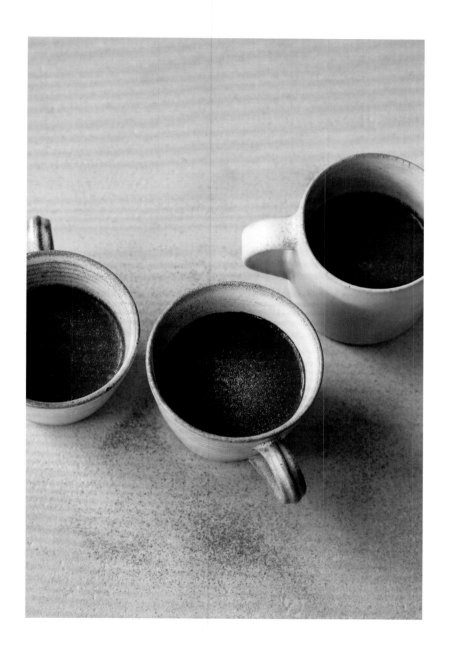

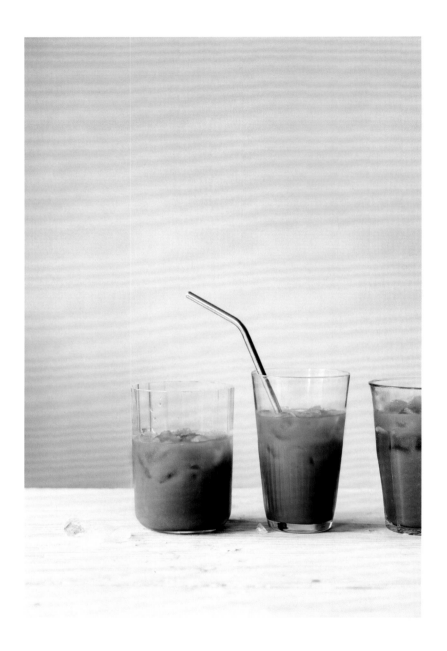

Drink your greens

I first made this for a client who didn't like to eat his greens. It took some tweaking to get it right, but this recipe was the winner. It is packed full of goodness but unlike other green juices actually tastes amazing – I probably have it at least once a week.

½ large cucumber, chopped
   into chunks
2 apples, cored and deseeded
5-cm piece of ginger
1 lime, peeled
20 mint leaves
1 small handful spinach
1 small handful kale
3–4 ice cubes

Pass the cucumber, apples, ginger and lime through an electric juicer. Pour the liquid into the jug of a powerful blender and add the mint leaves, spinach, kale and ice cubes. Blend for at least 1 minute on high or until the mixture is completely smooth. Pour into your serving glass over more ice, depending on how cold you would like it, and enjoy!

Pimp up your porridge

Serves 2

I've taken my grandma's recipe and given it a little pumping up for that extra 'wow' factor. It's a breakfast I'll make to load up before a big day, or to warm me up on a wintery morning. My dad might say his porridge is better as it's a classic Yorkshire favourite. But mine is obviously the best.

80g porridge oats
275ml oat milk
275ml water
½ tsp cinnamon
sweetener of your choice:
    honey/agave syrup/
    maple syrup

Peach and raspberry
100g raspberries
3 tbsp honey or syrup
1 ripe peach, stone removed and
    cut into slices
2 tbsp flaxseed
1 tbsp pistachios, finely chopped

Blueberry and coconut
100g blueberries
¼ tsp ground cardamom
1 tbsp chia seeds
3 tbsp honey or syrup
2 tbsp coconut flakes, toasted

Banana, date and pecan
60g dates, roughly chopped
3 tbsp honey or syrup
1 large ripe banana, thickly sliced
2 tbsp pecans, toasted and
    roughly chopped

Peach and raspberry

Place the oats, milk, water and cinnamon into a large saucepan. Add half of the raspberries and 1 tablespoon of honey or syrup to the oat mixture, and put over a high heat. Stir well and bring to the boil, then turn down to a simmer. Stir over a low heat for a few minutes until the porridge has thickened. Spoon into two bowls and top with the remaining raspberries. Add the peach slices, flaxseed and pistachios, and the rest of the honey or syrup.

Blueberry and coconut

Place the oats, milk, water and cinnamon into a large saucepan. Add half of the blueberries, the cardamom, chia seeds and 1 tablespoon of honey or syrup and put over a high heat. Stir well and bring to the boil, then turn it down to a simmer. Stir over a low heat for a few minutes until the porridge has thickened. Spoon into two bowls and top with the remaining blueberries, the coconut flakes and the rest of the honey or syrup.

Banana, date and pecan

Place the oats, milk, water and cinnamon into a large saucepan. Add half of the dates and 1 tablespoon of honey or syrup and put over a high heat. Stir well and bring to the boil, then turn it down to a simmer. Stir over a low heat for a few minutes until the porridge has thickened. Spoon into two bowls and top with the remaining dates, the sliced banana, pecans and the rest of the honey or syrup.

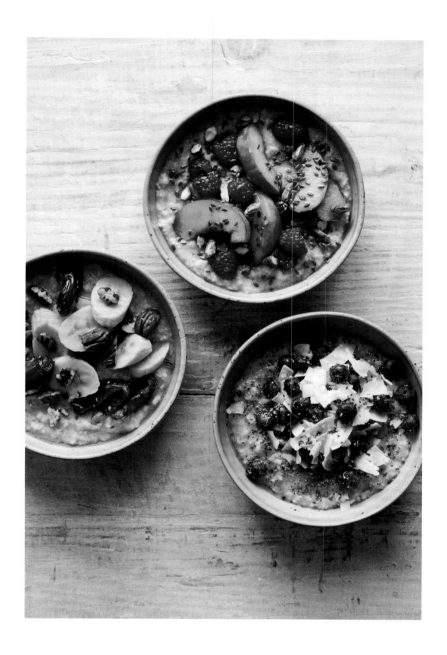

Fifteen-
minute
rituals

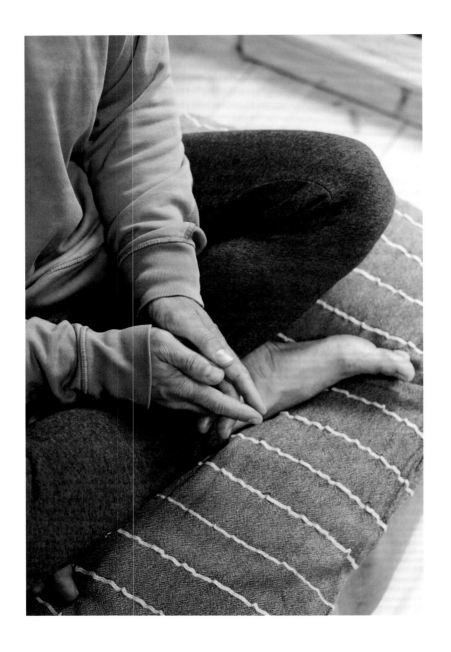

Your morning wake-up

We're combining breathing and mobility exercises here, for the ultimate calm and a focused start to the day. Think you haven't got fifteen minutes before the madness of the day begins? Set your alarm and get up earlier. I guarantee you won't regret it. Early rise, early vibes . . .

Start with five minutes of breathing

Sit on the side of the bed or somewhere comfortable and take a few purposeful breaths, deep into the belly. Remember to keep breathing through your nose if you can.

Now add a pause into your breath, which will give you focus and make you feel more awake and alert. Inhale for a count of four, hold for four, exhale for four, then hold again for four. Repeat until your five minutes is up. If a count of four feels too much, start with two or three and build it up slowly over several practices.

Ten minutes of movement

Once you've done this a few times and no longer need to look at the pictures, play with the movements and keep the flow going through the whole ten minutes. You'll feel warm, invigorated and ready to start the day.

If you're finding some of this hard, stay patient and keep practising. I couldn't have done all these movements before I started mobility training. Every time you mobilize your body, you make it stronger.

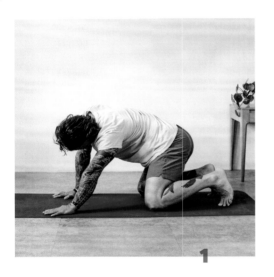
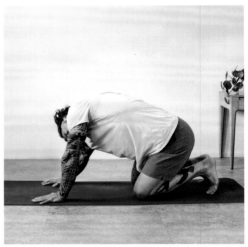

1

Start on all fours on your mat – wrists under shoulders, hips over knees, and toes tucked under. Begin with spinal articulation to mobilize your body, improve your range of motion, and set yourself up for the day: move your spine from side to side then backwards and forwards for one minute.

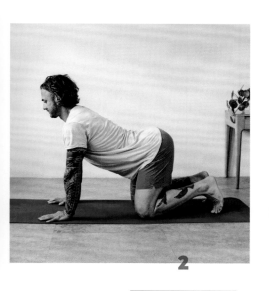

2

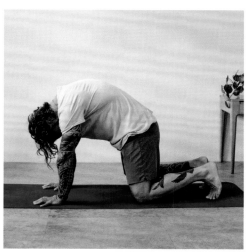

Now inhale as you lift your head up and tilt your hips back, arching your back. Breathe out and lift your spine to the sky, tucking your chin into your chest so that your back is rounded. Move between these two opposite stretches for one minute.

Repeat steps 1 and 2.

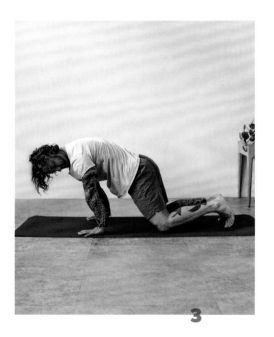

3

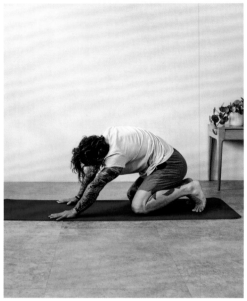

Next are free flow movements. Stay on all fours and move everything from the top of the head to the base of the spine and the hips. Get your shoulders and wrists going too. Really play with the movements and make them as fluid as you can.

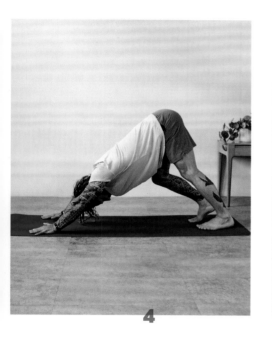

4

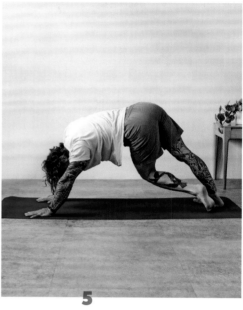

5

Now move into the downward dog position: spread your fingers, lift the hips towards the sky and tuck your chin into your chest. Do little walking movements with your feet, bending your knees if you need to. Feel the stretch in your Achilles tendon (at the back of your ankle), your calves and hamstrings.

Add a little twist now, bending one knee towards the centre of the mat and straightening the other leg so you feel a stretch in your hips and the side of the ribs. Do the same on the other side, then move back into downward dog.

Repeat steps 4 and 5.

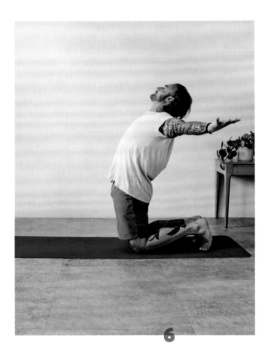

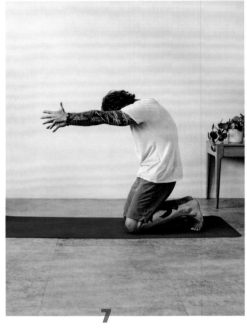

6

Push back to a kneeling position and sit up straight, pushing your hips forward and activating the gluteal muscles in your bottom. Lift your arms up in front of you, turning your palms to the ceiling so your thumbs are facing out. Inhale and swing your arms out to the side so you feel a stretch in the chest.

7

Breathe out and reach forwards, dropping your head slightly towards your chest and pushing your back away to open up the middle back.

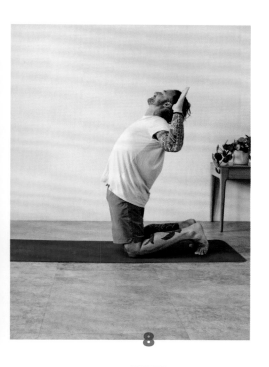

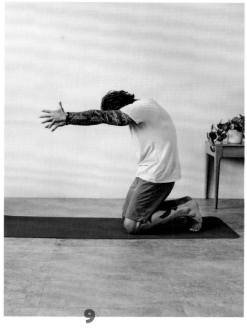

Inhale and bring your hands to side of your head, elbows bent, in the cactus position. Lean back slightly, opening your chest and stretching through the hips.

Breathe out and stretch your arms forwards as before, dropping the head and pushing your back away.

Cycle through steps 6–9 for two minutes.

10

Move to downward dog again, then step your left foot forwards so it's next to your left hand. Turn your right hand outwards, pushing the right heel back and towards the floor, activating the back leg. Move your left hand under your right shoulder and get the left elbow as near to the floor as you can as you sink deeper into your right hip. Let your left hip open and your left leg roll out a bit to help. You won't be able to master this immediately, but keep working at it. As your mobility improves, you'll get your elbow lower to the floor.

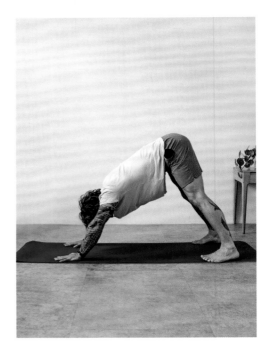

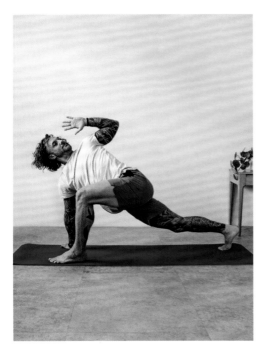

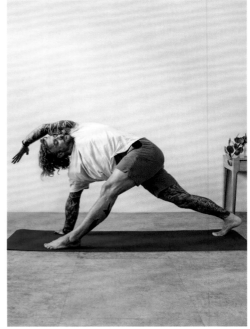

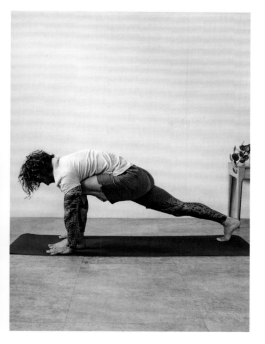

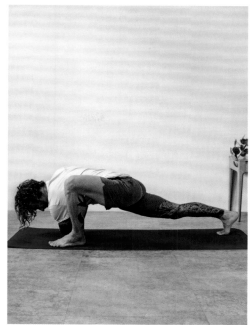

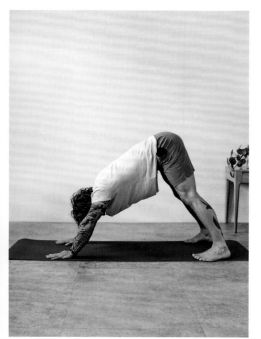

11

Inhale and then unravel your body to the left. Your right hand is still on the floor supporting you as the left arm moves across your body and into the air, so it is bent with the left hand by your left ear. Now straighten the left leg and stretch your left arm forwards to the front of the mat. Go back to downward dog, and repeat the exercise on the right side.

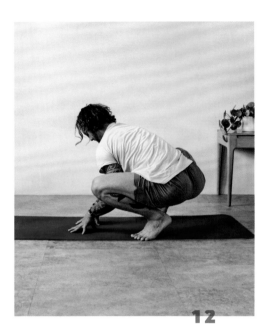

12

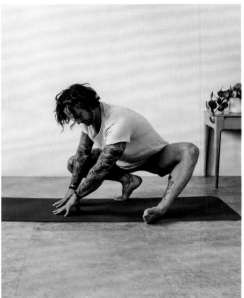

Now get into a squat position, feet wide and bottom low. Feel the stretch in your hip sockets for a few moments, then put your fingers on the floor in front of you and move from side to side a few times, working some gentle mobilization into the ankles and hips.

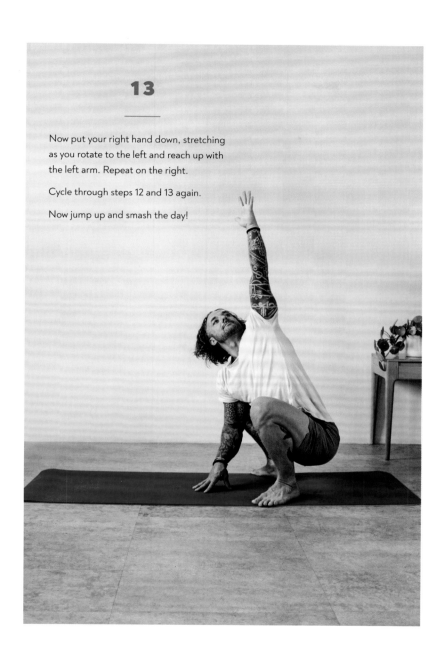

13

Now put your right hand down, stretching as you rotate to the left and reach up with the left arm. Repeat on the right.

Cycle through steps 12 and 13 again.

Now jump up and smash the day!

Audit your life
(and hold yourself to account)

It's easy to get caught up in a routine, whether that's your job, the food you're eating, or the time you're spending scrolling through social media or watching TV. Sometimes you need to catch yourself and ask: Is this making me happy? Am I living the life I really want and being the most productive I can be? Am I reaching the goals I have set for myself?

That's where a life audit comes in – taking fifteen minutes every month or so to check in with yourself and work out where you need to make changes.

Consider the areas of your life that are taking up headspace right now, and write down what's going well and what might need to change. Here are some questions to get you started:

- **What do you spend most of your day doing?** Is it a good use of your time, does it make you feel happy or is it something you want to change?
- **Are your relationships fulfilling?** Are there aspects of those relationships you want to improve?
- **Do you have a good balance between your work life,** home life and social life? Are there areas you can work on to improve the quality of connection and level of happiness?
- **Are you exercising enough,** getting outside, moving your body, and taking breaks to increase your focus and boost your creativity?
- **What's your diet like?** If you're being honest, have you noticed you've been snacking a little bit more and the number of sneaky treats has crept up? How has that made you feel?
- **How much time are you spending** in a phone vortex every day? Is the constant pinging of notifications distracting you?

Be brutally honest with yourself. Then, for each topic, write down a couple of practical changes that you know you could make. Keep them simple and achievable, otherwise you won't follow through.

To give you an example: if you don't like your job, is there something you can do about it, like suggesting a change to the work structure that might improve team communication or allow for more creativity? Or could you find time to get outside during the day to reset and refocus, and get some exercise in to stay energized? Or maybe you want to change direction in your career – is there a little side hustle you can work on in your spare time that will be a step in the right direction?

I do life audits every month – sometimes every week when life's a bit hectic. I write down what's working and what's not, and sometimes I make a list of pros and cons if I'm making a decision as a result. I would say audits are the key to me staying on track – they help me get rid of the stuff that no longer serves me, and make time for the things I really want to do.

A life audit can often take you down a path that feels uncomfortable – you may have to face things you would rather avoid, lean in to confrontation and make tough, challenging decisions. But I've never regretted doing one; I've always been happier after making the changes an audit leads to.

A key turning point for me was the life audit I carried out a few years after my injuries and lifestyle ended my rugby dream, when I'd gone off the rails. It was a tough time and I wasn't taking care of myself, either physically or mentally. I was eating junk food, drinking too much alcohol, not getting enough sleep and generally treating myself with very little respect. One day I looked at myself in the mirror, then wrote down what I needed to change. It was a harsh reality to face up to, seeing it written down in black and white. But I knew that if I wanted to survive and live a healthier life, something needed to change.

That audit may even have saved my life.

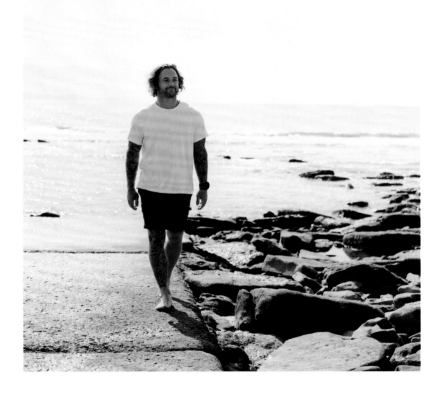

Good to know . . .
Scientists can tell from the pattern of your brain waves whether you're walking in green space or in built-up areas. They're calmer and less fired-up in green spaces.

A walking meditation

To some people, the idea of meditation can be off-putting. Perhaps you associate it with bendy men or women sitting cross-legged, and think it's not something for you. Perhaps it just seems too difficult, an unattainable state for your busy mind in its busy world.

If that's you – or if you've tried meditation before and not really got into it – a walking meditation can be a really good place to start, because you don't have to worry about sitting still or being 100 per cent focused.

What you are aiming for is to feel 'present' in the moment, rather than ruminating about the past or planning the future. It can be easier to achieve this presence while in motion because we can use walking's natural rhythm to help.

You can do a walking meditation either inside or outside. You don't need a lot of space, just enough room to take a few steps each way. Personally, I'd always choose to do it outside, because nature has the power to give an extra edge to your practice.

So, the first thing to do is check in. Stand still with your feet firmly anchored on the ground and your arms by your sides. Take note of your breath – in through the nose and out through the nose. Now try to take slightly fuller, deeper breaths.

Observe your surroundings, look down at your feet and hands, then gaze slowly at what's around you. Really open up your senses. Pause on what catches your eye, then tune back in to your breaths. Whenever you find your mind wandering, try to catch yourself and bring your attention back to your breathing, keeping it nice and steady.

Now start taking short, mindful steps around the space. Really slow it down, and try to pay attention to your body. Feel how your foot and leg leave the ground during each step, and how they reconnect with it as you place your foot back down. Feel the pressure of your soles on the ground.

You might stop every few steps, mindfully breathing in and out and observing any feelings and emotions you're having. Then pull yourself back to where you are physically and tune back into your breathing – has it changed? Try to keep your attention on the movement of your body. This isn't easy, and it will take some practice; every time you feel your mind wandering off, gently bring it back to your body and the here and now.

As you continue walking, notice the finest little details that are capturing your attention: a bird soaring, the wind moving the trees, a single blade of grass, the sounds (or silence) of your space. Take it in, watch it, and try to steady your breath even more.

If you're outside, concentrate on the ground beneath your feet. Maybe you're lucky enough to be able to have your bare feet in the grass or sand, and to really feel that connection to the earth.

When you have completed one circuit of your space, pause for a second or two, then start the process again and keep going until fifteen minutes are up.

Whatever the weather, walking in nature has been shown to be good for keeping your heart healthy and your fitness levels topped up. And according to a gazillion studies over the years, it has measurable mental benefits as well. It may even reduce the risk of those depressive states that seem to be running rife in too many lives. We sometimes just need a friendly reminder to get up and get out. This is mine to you . . .

A cold shower

If this doesn't sound like too much fun, bear with me. Since training to be a Master Coach at XPT (Extreme Performance Training) in California, I have witnessed first-hand the incredible benefits of an ice bath. Immersion in icy-cold water is a key pillar of the XPT lifestyle: it can speed up your recovery after physical exertion, reduces swelling and inflammation, and wow does it invigorate you.

But the really interesting thing for me is the mental resilience that the exposure to cold water can give you – and I'm not just talking elite athletes, but anyone wanting to improve their ability to deal with and adapt to stress.

By shocking your body but learning to remain calm, you are building up your confidence that you can withstand this temporary discomfort and come out the other side unscathed. That will translate into being more resilient in everyday life when faced with stress – whether that's an argument with your boss, a driver shouting at you in traffic, or an impossible deadline.

A cold shower can also alter your brain chemistry. One study showed it massively increased levels of the feel-good brain chemicals noradrenaline and dopamine, which can give you positive energy and an increased sense of optimism. In another intriguing study, a group of people switched their warm shower to cold for a few seconds. They did this every day for several weeks, and it had a significant antidepressive effect.

To start with, I suggest turning a warm fifteen-minute shower to the cold setting for the last thirty seconds or so. Pretty much every muscle and cell in your body will scream out in protest, but here's what you do:

- **Go immediately to your breath** to calm yourself down. Breathe more slowly than usual and take deeper breaths, aiming to exhale for longer than the inhalation. So, inhale for three and exhale for five, to calm your system.
- **Sit with that feeling of discomfort** for a few moments while continuing your

breath practice. Feel how your body is overcoming the distress and returning to its baseline.

- **Step out and get warm!**

Don't stay too long under a cold shower. If you are shivering, you have probably pushed yourself too far. What this exercise is about is learning to manage the stress before you cross that boundary. Play with the edge of it, and build up your tolerance gradually.

Once you can cope with thirty seconds of cold, try increasing it incrementally up to about ninety seconds. You won't always be able to stay under it that long. I have been practising ice and cold therapy for years now, and a cold shower still gets me. Sometimes I can stay in it for a few minutes, and other times it's only ten seconds – it really depends on my mood and headspace that day.

If you prefer, you can alternate warm and cold water during your shower: maybe ten seconds of cold, then turn the shower off or step out of the water and steady the nervous system response; then twenty seconds of warm, and keep switching. Observe your experience and try to find the upper limit of your tolerance while staying calm. It's a powerful practice.

If you are on medication or are particularly susceptible to shocks or triggers (whether physical or mental), you may want to consult your doctor before trying this one out.

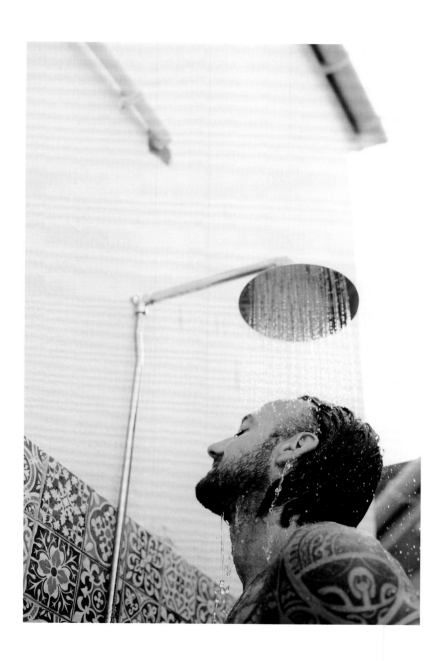

My ultimate bedtime flow

Use this to down-regulate after a workout or to prepare your body for bed, stretching away the tensions of the day. Keep the movements calm and slower than usual, really feeling each stretch.

Start with some breaths – nice and deep, in and out through the nose. Add a pause after you inhale, then exhale, making the out-breath as long and steady as you can. Practise this for a couple of minutes, and try to use this same cadence of breathing throughout the flow, keeping the exhale longer than the inhale. This will calm and relax you.

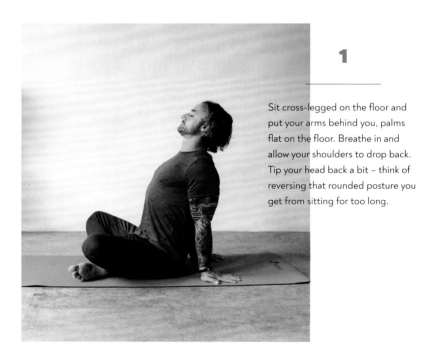

1

Sit cross-legged on the floor and put your arms behind you, palms flat on the floor. Breathe in and allow your shoulders to drop back. Tip your head back a bit – think of reversing that rounded posture you get from sitting for too long.

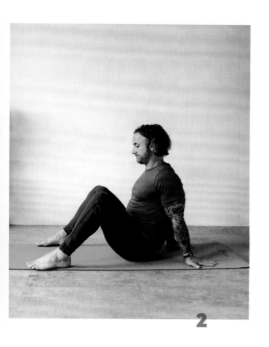
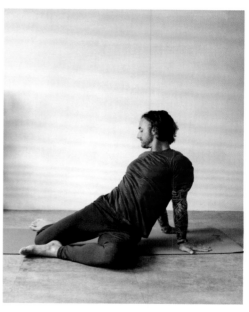

2

Uncross your legs and place your feet wide (a little more than hip distance apart). With your knees bent, drop them to the left, rolling your hips and putting just a tiny bit of force into pushing the top leg towards the floor so you can feel the stretch in your hip. Hold the stretch for a few moments and then do the same thing on the right. Repeat several times.

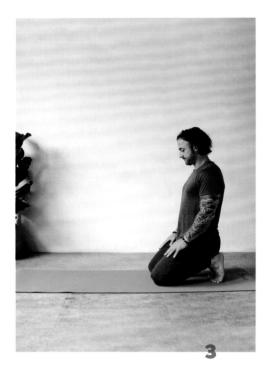
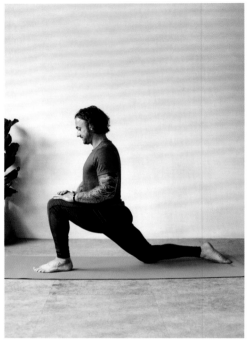

3

Get onto your knees and step forwards with the left leg, knee bent. Gently lean forwards into that left knee, hands on top of the thigh. Don't force it, but try to feel a stretch in your right quad (the front of your thigh). Work through a few stretches backwards and forwards with this movement, allowing the right hip to open when you move forwards and dropping the pelvis slightly. Try to keep your upper body fairly straight.

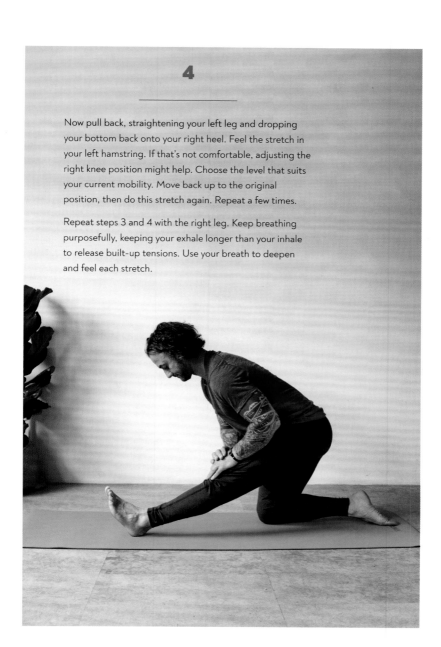

4

Now pull back, straightening your left leg and dropping your bottom back onto your right heel. Feel the stretch in your left hamstring. If that's not comfortable, adjusting the right knee position might help. Choose the level that suits your current mobility. Move back up to the original position, then do this stretch again. Repeat a few times.

Repeat steps 3 and 4 with the right leg. Keep breathing purposefully, keeping your exhale longer than your inhale to release built-up tensions. Use your breath to deepen and feel each stretch.

5

Go onto all fours, then slowly lift your hips into the air, straightening your legs into a downward dog pose, pushing away from the floor. Hold for a few moments, then drop your knees to the floor, under the hips. Stretch your arms out in front of you – palms to the floor, fingers nice and wide – and drop your chest to the floor, your hips moving back. Feel your back opening up. Stay like this for a few breath cycles, or longer if you want.

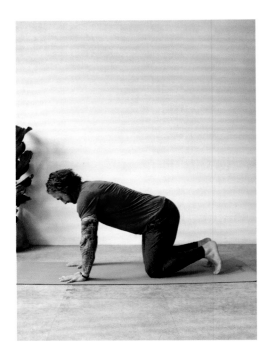

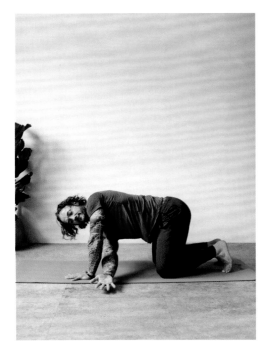

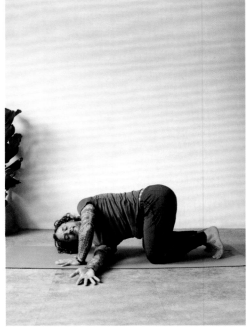

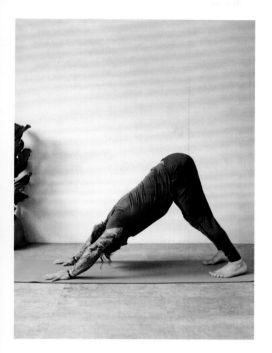 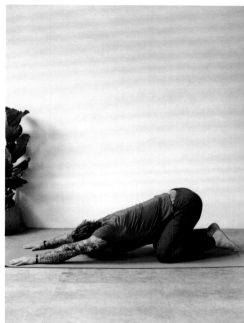

6

Inhale and return to all fours. On the exhale, reach across with your right arm and thread it under your body, past your left wrist, twisting your body and dropping your right shoulder and your head to the mat. Hold for a few moments, then inhale and repeat on the other side.

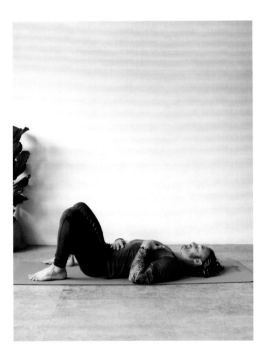
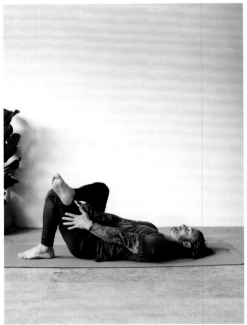

7

Lie with your back on the mat, knees bent. Really concentrate for a minute of slow and deliberate breathing, with nice long exhales. Now cross the right ankle over the left knee. Pull on your left thigh with both hands, keeping the pressure level so your right shin stays more or less parallel to the ground. Rock gently left to right several times.

Now spread your arms out on the floor, and make the movement bigger: the right foot should put pressure on your left knee, so you feel the opening in the right hip and hopefully a nice release in the lower back. When you twist over to the left you can press your knee with your left hand if it feels good.

Repeat for the other side.

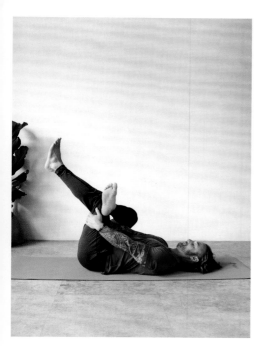
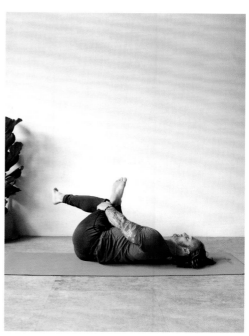
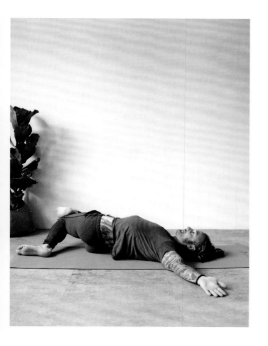
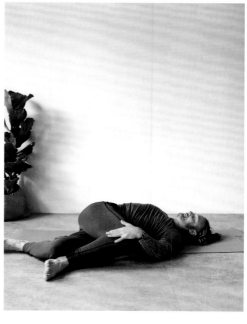

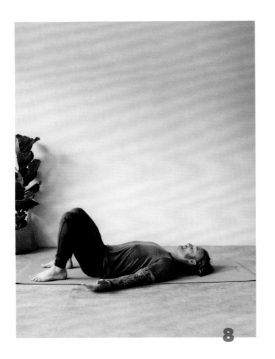
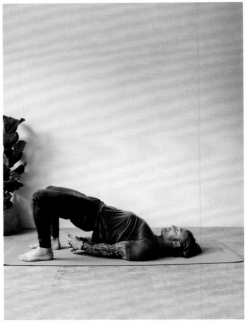

8

Return to a knees-bent position, still lying down. Inhale and raise your hips off the floor. Now 'walk' up onto your shoulder blades so you're in a bridge position. Interlock your fingers under your body, bringing the elbows towards each other, or put your hands on the floor if you prefer. Hold the stretch. Then move your hands back to the floor and lower your hips back down.

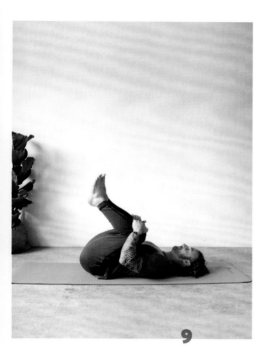

9

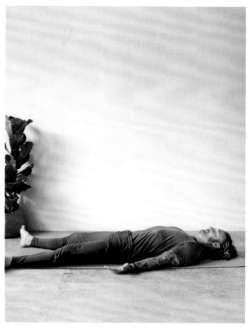

Hug your knees to your chest, take your tailbone off the floor and gently rock from side to side, opening the knees slightly. Finish by lying flat on the mat, letting your legs and arms relax and roll out. Breathe steadily in and out several times, and really ground yourself on the mat. Now you're good to chill. Sleep well!

Insomnia rescue

If you can't sleep, lying in bed at 3 a.m. trying to force yourself to sleep never works. It is better to get up, go to another room and do some calming breathing and movement practices.

Try sitting or lying somewhere comfortable and simply observe your breathing: take a steady breath in and out again through the nose. Make the exhalation a little longer than the inhale to stimulate the body's relaxation response. If your mind is super-stimulated, add a pause after the inhale and before the exhalation. Repeat the cycle and continue for a few minutes. If your mind starts to wander, bring your attention back to your breath. If you're feeling sleepy now, head back to bed and keep that breathing pattern until you drift off. If not, try these ten gentle movements:

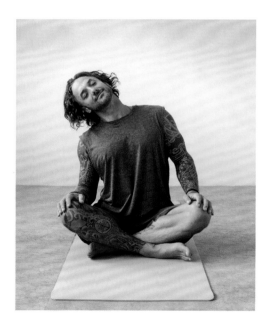

1

Sit on the floor, legs crossed or out in front of you, and tip your head from left to right and back again a few times, then forwards and back, to stretch the neck. Keep the movement super slow: imagine you are moving in a jar of honey, as my yoga teacher used to say. Find a nice fluid flow as you move your neck and progress to your shoulders, while keeping the same long-exhalation breath pattern mentioned above. If you find a spot in your neck or shoulders that might be holding a bit of tension, pause and stay with it for a few moments while you breathe out.

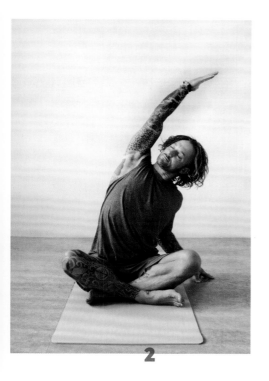

2

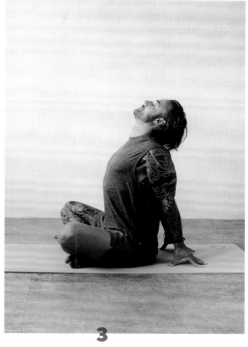

3

Put your left hand down on the floor next to you and reach over your head with your right arm, bending the head towards the floor and stretching through the right side of the body. Do the same on the other side.

Put your hands on the floor slightly behind you, opening up the chest and squeezing your shoulder blades together as you lean your head back. Hold that stretch for a few moments.

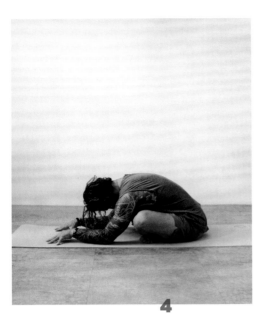

4

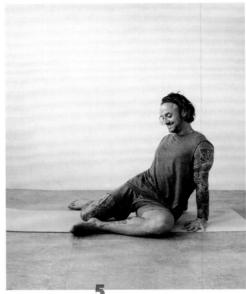

5

Uncross your legs and fold yourself forwards, letting your head hang down towards your knees. Hold for a few moments.

Place your feet flat on the floor, knees bent, and drop your knees from side to side to release the tension in your hips. Keep these movements really slow.

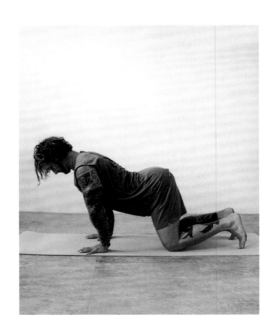

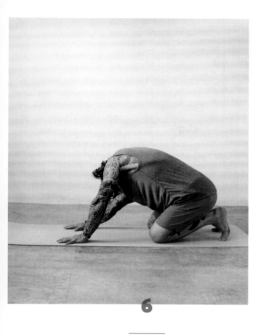

6

Move to all fours and do some gentle
spinal articulation, moving your hips
and spine, left to right and up and down,
loosening up your back.

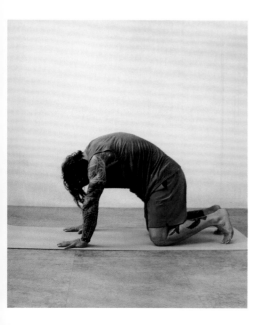

7

Inhale as you arch your back, tilting your
pelvis back so your tailbone sticks up
(cow stretch). Exhale as you tuck your chin
into your chest, dropping your head and
rounding your spine towards the ceiling,
pushing the mat away (cat stretch).
Cycle through the cat and cow stretches
a few times.

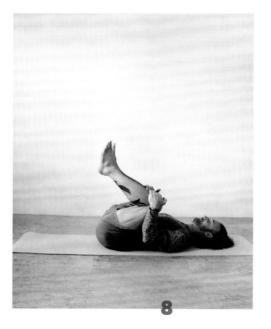

8

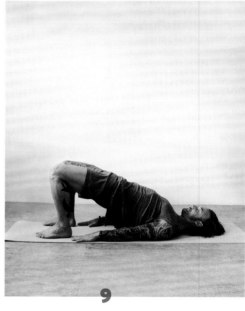

9

Lie on your back, knees bent, and rock your body left to right and back again. Repeat this a few times.

With your feet flat on the floor, lift your hips up and 'walk' up onto your shoulder blades in a gentle bridge position. Place your arms either side of you on the floor and push into the feet.

Lower yourself down and rock the legs and knees left and right. Hug your knees to your chest.

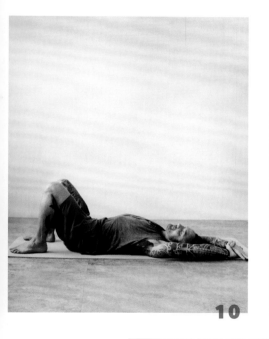
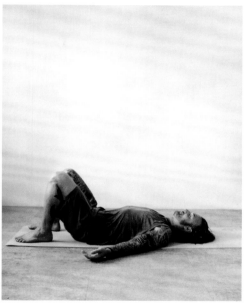

Still lying down, stretch your arms overhead on the floor and grab your right wrist with your left hand gently pulling to the left. Hold for a few moments, then change sides.

After you've completed the ten steps, finish by lying down, arms resting on the floor at a forty-five-degree angle to your body, and do a final breath practice: inhale for three, hold for three, exhale for six. Take as much time as you need here, but a good target is ten full breathing cycles.

By now you should be ready to head back to bed. Keep that final breath practice going as you lie in bed, and it won't be long before you're drifting off to sleep.

"

Health habits don't need to take up your whole day or involve anything complicated. Concentrate on getting the basics right and apply them to your day when you can fit them in – and you will see them transform the way your body feels and your mind behaves. Breathe mindfully, move slowly, take the time you need to heal and repair. Then you will be capable of applying that power to anything else in your life.

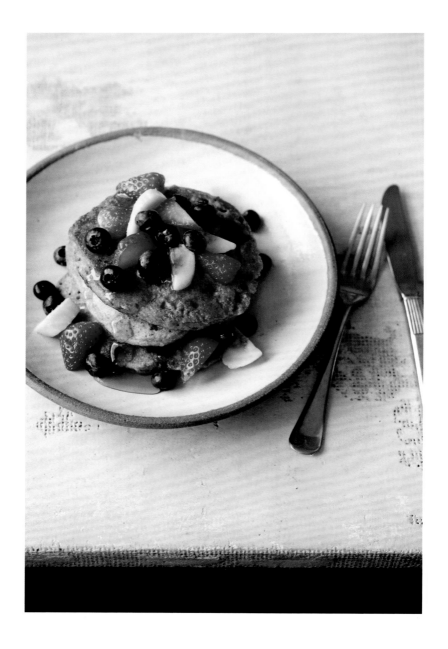

Maple and banana berry pancakes

When I make this I'm reminded of my first adventures in America, when I was playing rugby and filling my face with stacks of pancakes most mornings to load up. Over the years it's fair to say I've sampled a few different combos, and this recipe is one of my favourites.

180g self-raising wholemeal flour
1 tsp baking powder
½ tsp ground cinnamon
1 large free-range egg
1 tsp vanilla extract
¾ large banana, mashed
230ml oat milk
1 tbsp maple syrup (or sweetener of choice)
2 tbsp desiccated coconut, toasted
50g blueberries
2 tsp vegetable oil
20g butter

Toppings
200g mixed berries
¼ large banana, sliced
maple syrup to serve

Place the flour, baking powder and cinnamon into a mixing bowl. Add the egg, vanilla extract, mashed banana, oat milk and tablespoon of maple syrup (or your alternative), and whisk until smooth.

Fold in the coconut and blueberries. Heat a large non-stick frying pan over a medium-high heat. Add half the oil and half the butter, and wait for it to melt.

Put large spoonfuls of pancake batter into the pan. You can choose how big to make your pancakes, depending on the size of your pan. (I like to do four at a time.) Cook for 1 minute, or until a few little bubbles begin to appear on the top of each pancake. Flip over and cook for a further 1–2 minutes.

Repeat with the remaining batter and stack the pancakes on plates to serve. Top with the mixed berries and your remaining sliced banana and slather in maple syrup (or your sweetener of choice).

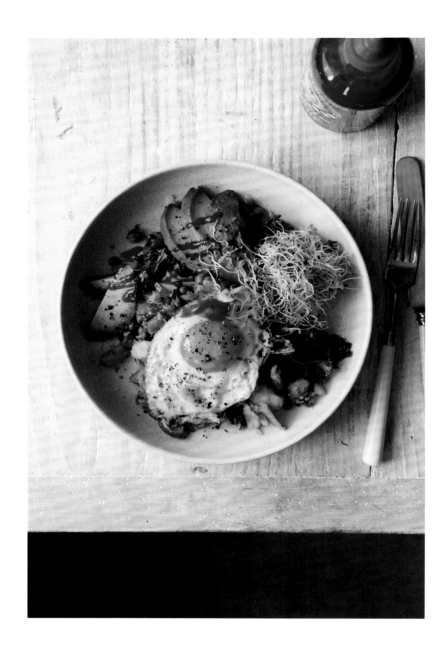

Leftover smash hash

Serves 2

Another Yorkshire fave, this is ideal for when you don't want to let any of the leftovers go to waste after a big feast – or for those times you need to clear the fridge and get creative. I think the leftovers from a big roast dinner often taste better the next day anyway, but this is a recipe that will make your belly smile any day of the week.

400g leftover roast veg
(pumpkin, parsnip, potatoes, brussel sprouts, onion, sweet potato)
2 tbsp butter (or dairy-free spread)
2 tsp olive oil
2 large free-range eggs
1 large handful frozen peas
2 large handfuls kale
1 tbsp fresh sage, finely chopped
½ ripe avocado, sliced
1 large handful alfalfa sprouts (see p. 264)
2 tbsp sriracha sauce

Lightly mash up your veg with a fork. Whatever leftover roast veg you have can work here.

Place a large non-stick frying pan over a high heat. Add half the butter and half the olive oil. When the pan is hot and the butter is sizzling, add the leftover veg and leave to cook for a few minutes, without stirring the pan. This helps you get a crispy edge on the veg.

Meanwhile, heat the remaining olive oil and butter in a medium frying pan. When the butter is melted, crack the eggs in and season well with salt and pepper. Cook the eggs for 3–4 minutes.

Now stir the leftover veg and add the frozen peas, kale and sage. Cook for a further 2 minutes. Season well and divide between two plates. Top each plate with a fried egg, avocado slices, alfalfa sprouts and sriracha.

Asian vegetable noodle soup

LUNCH   Serves 2

A staple part of my week is an Asian-inspired bowl of goodness. I'll vary it quite a bit, but I can never go wrong with mixing some extra veggies in with the noodles and adding some spice – it always hits the spot.

1.2 litres vegetable stock
2-cm piece of ginger, finely sliced or julienned
2 garlic cloves, sliced
2 kaffir lime leaves, finely shredded (see p. 265)
1 medium carrot, diced
6 baby corn, sliced
100g courgette, diced
75g cauliflower, roughly chopped
75g tenderstem broccoli, roughly chopped
2 egg noodle nests, broken up into smaller pieces
1 tbsp light soy sauce
2 tsp sesame oil
1 handful coriander, roughly chopped
1 red chilli, finely sliced

Put the stock, ginger, garlic and kaffir lime leaves into a medium saucepan. Put over a high heat and bring to the boil.

Add the carrot and corn and cook for 3 minutes before adding the courgette, cauliflower and broccoli. Cook for 2 minutes and then add the noodles. Reduce the heat to a simmer, then add the soy sauce and half the sesame oil. Cook for a further 4 minutes, or until the noodles are soft.

Stir in half the coriander and ladle into two large bowls, then drizzle with the remaining sesame oil. Top with the rest of the coriander and the chilli.

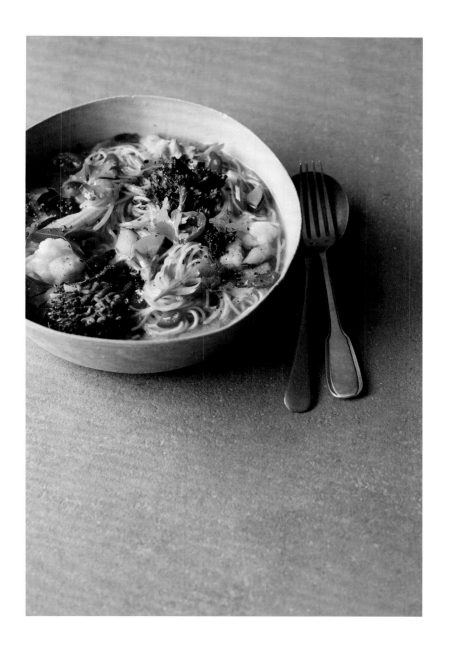

Kimchi and greens brown rice bowl

LUNCH

Serves 2

I literally lived off this little bowl of magic while backpacking in Thailand. It was super-cheap and always did the trick when I wanted a quick and easy meal. Now it transports me back to those adventures where my love of Asian food first began.

2 tbsp vegetable oil
250g smoked tofu, cut into 2-cm cubes
100g chestnut mushrooms, quartered
80g green beans, trimmed and halved
1 garlic clove, finely chopped
1 tsp gochujang (optional)
50ml water
250g cooked brown rice
100g kimchi, roughly chopped (see p. 265)
3 baby pak choi, roughly chopped
1 tbsp light soy sauce
1 tsp sesame oil
2 large free-range eggs

Garnish
50g kimchi
1 long red chilli, finely sliced
2 spring onions, finely sliced on the angle
furikake to sprinkle (see p. 264)

Heat a medium non-stick sauté pan or wok over a high heat. When hot, add half the vegetable oil and the tofu cubes and cook for 2 minutes, or until they are browned all over. Next add the mushrooms, green beans and garlic, and stir-fry for 1 minute.

Put in the gochujang and stir well for 1 minute, before adding the water and rice. Keep stirring for 2 minutes. Add the kimchi, pak choi, soy sauce and sesame oil, and stir-fry for a further 3 minutes.

Meanwhile, heat a small frying pan over a high heat. When hot, add the remaining vegetable oil and crack in the eggs. Season with salt and pepper and cook for 3 minutes, or until crispy on the bottom.

Divide the rice mixture between two bowls. Top each with a fried egg, and garnish with kimchi, chilli and spring onions. Sprinkle a little furikake over each one and enjoy.

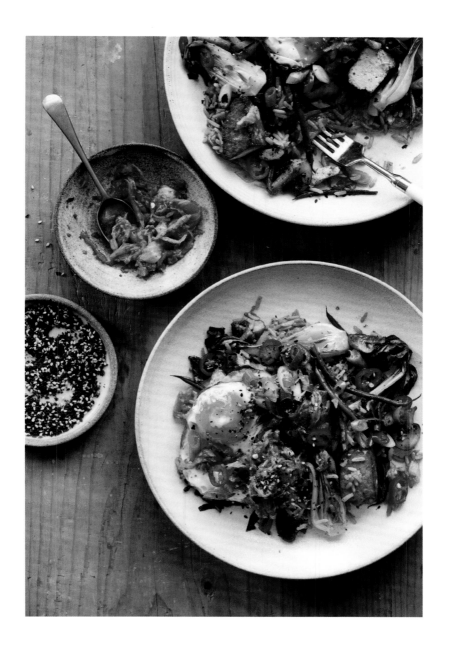

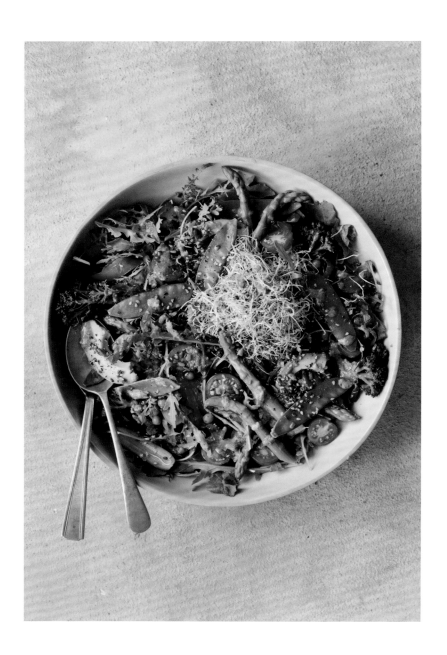

Midday munch for the mind

LUNCH

Serves 2

This does what it says on the tin – it's fully loaded with nutrients, flavour and crunch. Light on the digestive system, this will still fill you up and keep you sharp and satisfied for a few hours.

75g asparagus spears, trimmed
75g tenderstem broccoli, trimmed
4 baby courgettes, halved lengthwise
60g frozen peas, defrosted
2 large handfuls rocket
60g mangetout
8 cherry tomatoes, halved
60g roasted peppers, sliced
½ avocado, sliced
1 large handful alfalfa sprouts (see p. 264)
2 tbsp savoury seeds, toasted (see p. 265)

Dressing
1 heaped tsp Dijon mustard
1 tsp pesto
2 tbsp extra-virgin olive oil
1 tbsp sherry vinegar (or red wine vinegar)

Cut the asparagus spears in half and add to a sauté pan along with the broccoli, courgette and 50ml water. Season with salt and pepper and place the pan over a medium-high heat. Stir well until the water has evaporated and the vegetables are just cooked. Remove from the heat and stir in the peas.

Add a handful of rocket to the bottom of your bowl. Top with the mangetout and cherry tomatoes. Add the cooked vegetables, roasted pepper and avocado.

Mix the dressing ingredients together and spoon over the top. Sprinkle with sprouts and seeds and get involved!

Chinese-style smoked tofu and veggie stir-fry

Serves 2

Takeaways were a big part of my youth, but I realized a few years ago that you can make them at home just as fast, and they're much tastier and healthier . . . stir-fries have been a game-changer ever since. It's a rapid, light and healthy meal that's packed full of goodness, with all the colours and all the crunch.

2 tsp Chinese fermented black beans (or 100– 120ml pre-made black bean sauce)
2 tbsp boiling water (for the beans)
1 tbsp vegetable oil
250g smoked tofu, cubed
75g carrot, thinly sliced
6 baby corn, halved
2 garlic cloves, finely chopped
2-cm piece of ginger, finely chopped
100g baby chestnut mushrooms, halved
½ red pepper, sliced
75g tenderstem broccoli
100ml veg stock or water
100g mangetout and sugar snap mix
120g pak choi, cut into 8-cm lengths
75g edamame beans
2 tbsp shaoxing rice wine (see p. 266)
1½ tbsp light soy sauce
2 tsp sesame oil
1 tsp cornflour, mixed with 1–2 tbsp water

Place the black beans and boiling water into a small bowl. Once the beans have softened slightly, lightly mash them with the back of a teaspoon. (Ignore this step if you are using a pre-made sauce.)

Next, place a small wok or sauté pan over a high heat. When it is smoking hot, add the vegetable oil and tofu cubes, and stir-fry until they have browned on all sides. Next, add the carrot and baby corn and cook for a further 2 minutes. Stir in the garlic and ginger and cook for 1 minute before adding the mushrooms, pepper and tenderstem broccoli. Add the vegetable stock or water along with the black beans, and cook for another 3–4 minutes, then stir in the mangetout and sugar snap mix, pak choi and edamame beans. Pour in the shaoxing, soy sauce and sesame oil.

When everything is cooked, add the cornflour and water mixture. Stir quickly and remove from the heat. Serve in two bowls and enjoy!

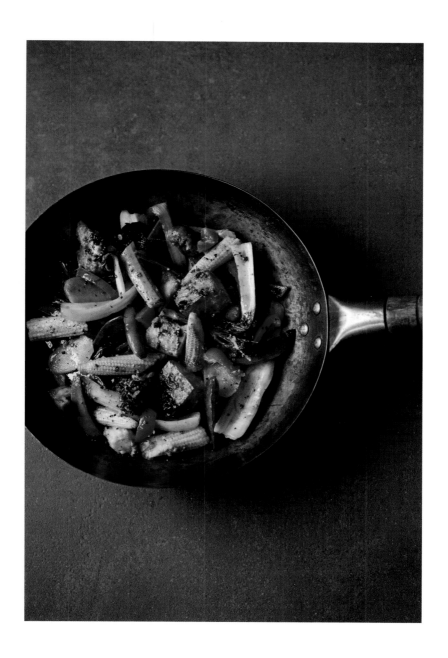

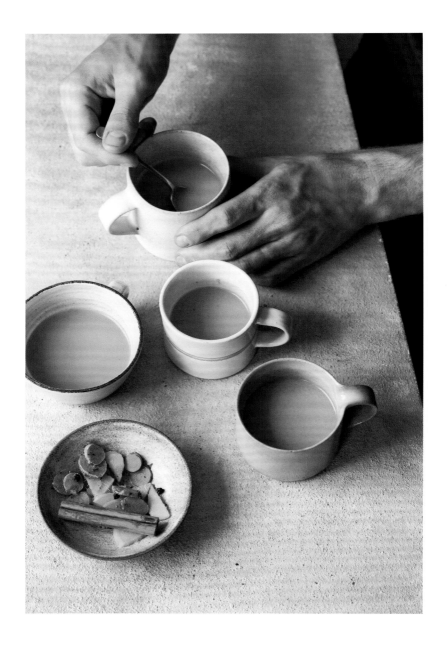

Golden turmeric

DRINKS

Serves 2

Another part of my yoga journey is this soothing golden cup of love. One of my fellow teachers showed me a recipe she had found in India, to which she'd added some extra spices to give it more of a kick. Now the legend lives on in this book, with a little Richie magic.

500ml coconut milk
8-cm piece of fresh turmeric, thinly sliced (or 1 tsp ground turmeric)
2.5-cm piece of ginger, thinly sliced
1 cinnamon stick, broken
2 cardamom pods, lightly smashed
6 peppercorns, lightly crushed
1 tbsp honey
2 tsp bee pollen

Put the coconut milk, turmeric, ginger, cinnamon stick, cardamom and peppercorns into a small saucepan. Place the saucepan over a low heat and gently bring up to a simmer (this should take about 5 minutes). Next, lower the heat so that the mixture is at a very gentle simmer, and let it cook for another 10 minutes, stirring occasionally.

Taste a little of the mixture at this point, and add the honey according to how sweet you like it. Strain the mixture through a sieve into a jug. If you prefer it frothy, pour the mixture into a blender and whizz for a couple of minutes before pouring into mugs. Sprinkle with a little bee pollen and serve.

Peanut butter and walnut cookies

Makes 12 cookies

Be warned – if you already have an addiction to cookies (and nut butter), these are next level and packed with energy to keep you going for hours. They're super-easy to make too, so all the family can get involved. (Thank me later!)

50g rolled oats
50g toasted walnuts,
    roughly chopped
50g dark chocolate chips
50g light muscovado sugar
pinch salt
75g self-raising flour
1 large free-range egg,
    lightly beaten
1 tsp vanilla extract
100g crunchy peanut butter

Preheat the oven to 190°C/170°C fan/Gas Mark 5.

Put the oats, walnuts, chocolate chips, muscovado sugar, salt and self-raising flour into a medium bowl. Mix these ingredients together well.

Add the beaten egg, vanilla extract and crunchy peanut butter, and mix thoroughly so that the ingredients all come together into a rough dough.

Divide the cookie mixture into 12 evenly sized balls. Flatten each one in your hands and then place onto a greaseproof-paper-lined baking tray. Leave at least 2 centimetres of space between each cookie.

Bake in the oven for 10 minutes, or until slightly browned. Remove, and leave to cool slightly on the tray. These are delicious when eaten still warm, perhaps with a glass of cold milk or a cup of tea or coffee.

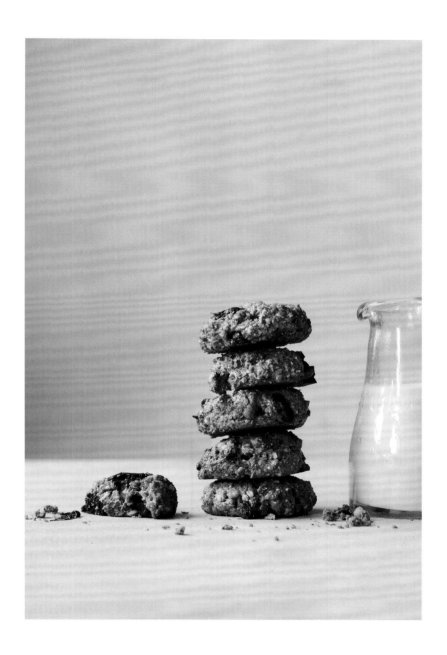

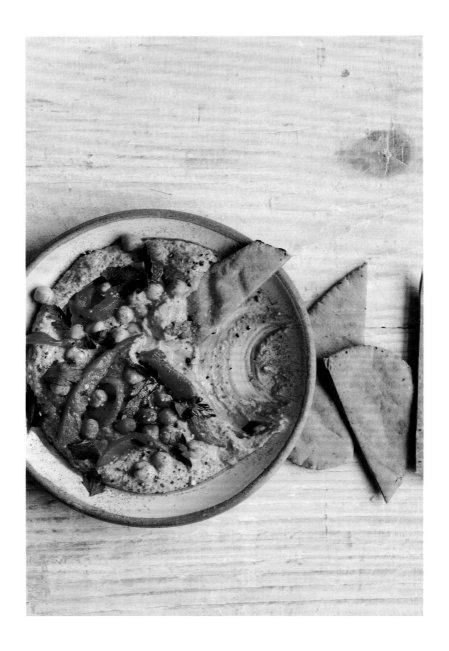

Smoky red pepper hummus

Serves 6–8

Simple and fast to prep, this hummus is perfect for snack time when hosting friends or for a solo dipping feast. This is my go-to healthy snack to help tide me over and keep my tummy satisfied between meals.

1 tbsp olive oil
3 garlic cloves, thickly sliced
1 onion, diced
1 tsp sweet smoked paprika
1 tsp ground cumin
2 x 400g cans chickpeas
200g roasted red peppers
    (from a jar), chopped
juice of 1 lemon
2 tbsp tahini
40ml extra-virgin olive oil

Garnish
1 tbsp extra-virgin olive oil
1 tsp flat-leaf parsley,
    finely chopped
pinch smoked paprika

Heat 1 tablespoon of olive oil in a small frying pan over a medium heat. Add the garlic and onion and cook for 4 minutes, or until they are softened and beginning to brown. Next, stir through the smoked paprika and cumin, along with a little salt, and remove from the heat.

Empty the two cans of chickpeas along with their liquid into a small saucepan. Put this over a medium heat and bring up to a gentle simmer for about 5 minutes, or until the chickpeas are warmed through. Remove from the heat and drain the chickpeas through a sieve, making sure to keep the warm chickpea liquid.

Place the onion mixture into a jug blender or food processor. Add the roasted red peppers and chickpeas (removing 2 tablespoons of chickpeas and 2 tablespoons of peppers for the garnish), then add the lemon juice, tahini, extra-virgin olive oil and 2 tablespoons of the chickpea water. Blend until smooth, adding more of the water if you need to, and season with salt and pepper to taste. Transfer the mixture to a container and place in the fridge to cool for an hour, or until you are ready to serve.

To serve, spoon the hummus into a large bowl and make a divot in the centre. Place the peppers you set aside in the centre along with the remaining chickpeas. Pour in 1 tablespoon of extra-virgin olive oil and sprinkle with flat-leaf parsley and smoked paprika. Serve with toasted pita bread and crudités.

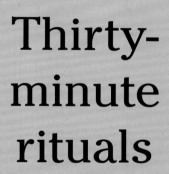

Thirty-minute rituals

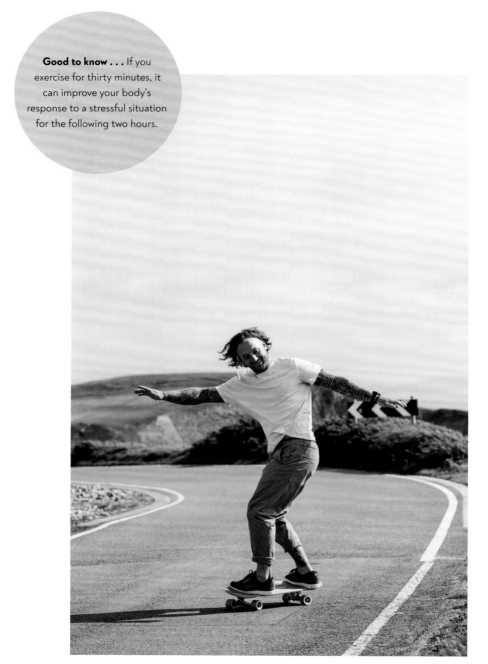

A mini adventure

If you want to give both your body and your brain a little love and TLC today, there is really no better way than getting outside for half an hour (or more, ideally) and simply moving your bum.

OK, it might be dark and cold when you finally find a gap in your day, or maybe the kids need you, or you're not feeling very energetic, or perhaps the dog ate your trainers? Whatever your reason for not getting out there, I promise you: getting outside in nature every day is a game-changer for body and mind. You just have to take the first step.

Some ideas for your mini adventure:
- **Get on your bike.** Have a quick look at a map, pick a direction to go in, and go explore.
- **Walk up a hill,** and get that heart pumping.
- **Take the kids to the park** and join in their fun, rather than sitting on a bench on your phone.
- **Discover a local footpath** you didn't know about, and see where it goes.
- **Take a walk in the woods.** The Japanese call this *shinrin-yoku* ('forest bathing'); walking among trees lowers blood pressure and stress hormone levels, and boosts the body's immune system.
- **Run a new route.** If you're not that into running or you're new to it, start with a high-low option: one minute of running; four minutes at a walk.

Exercising puts you in a positive frame of mind wherever you do it, but doing it outside in nature is a super power-up for your mental and physical health. In fact, science tells us that 'green exercise' has multiple benefits:
- **It revitalizes you** and keeps your spirits up.
- **It keeps anger,** tension and depressive feelings in check.
- **It improves your confidence** and self-esteem.

- **Outdoor exercise** is more satisfying and enjoyable than exercise indoors.
- **It increases your ability** to deal with life's stresses.
- **It helps tune your body clock** so you sleep better – especially when you do it in the morning.
- **Exercising outdoors** helps you get your vitamin D dose for the day (between April and October in the UK).

Be more wild – it's part of being human. Be in nature, get lost in nature, explore nature. After all, we are nature.

Personally, I wouldn't have made it this far without the connection I feel with the ocean and nature – especially when I'm surfing, hiking or riding a bike. The peace and calm and headspace that nature has given me over the years when the world has felt pretty lonely and dark has been immense – whether I'm playing in it or just quietly sitting, immersed in it . . .

So just get out and feel! 'It's good for your mind, body and soul' (said a very wise and happy hippy). If you don't believe me, why not try something new this week and take yourself on a little adventure? I challenge you . . .

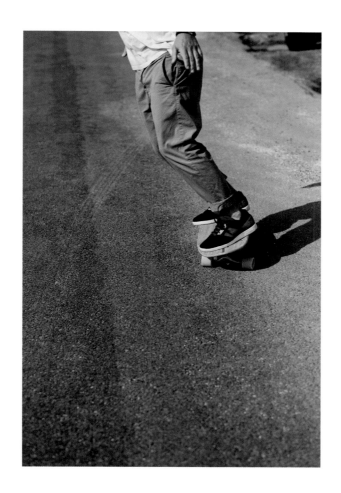

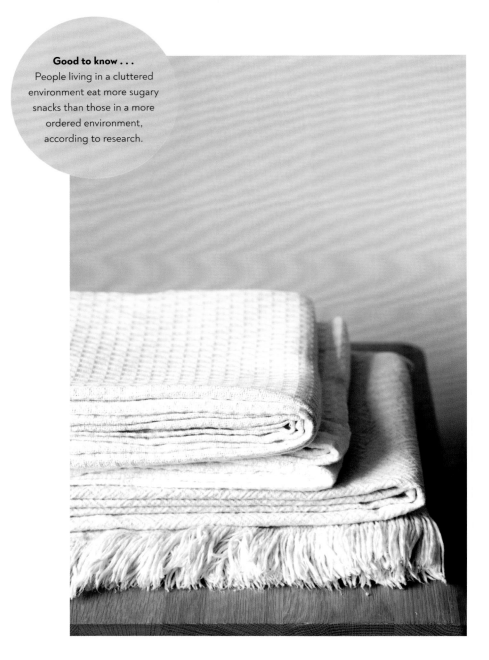

Good to know . . .

People living in a cluttered environment eat more sugary snacks than those in a more ordered environment, according to research.

Clear space, clear mind

I'm living proof that taking just a little bit of time to clear your space can . . . clear your headspace too. Creating more order and harmony in your home can make you feel more alive, more focused, and generally more in control of that distractible monkey mind.

I find that when I devote a bit of time to decluttering, I create more time for the things I want to achieve – because I'm not distracted or overwhelmed by the mess around me.

And it's not just me. There's solid evidence from science that living in a cluttered, chaotic environment can distract your brain by bombarding it with too many visual stimuli so it can't focus properly. It can also cause your stress hormone levels to rise, and sap the motivation you need for what's really important.

Getting rid of clutter can:
- **Give you a feel-good rush.**
- **Increase your motivation.**
- **Decrease stress** and make you less irritable.
- **Improve your cognitive powers.**
- **Make you feel calm** and more in control.

The process is where the magic happens. You might find a hidden treasure you completely forgot about. You might also be able to work through your feelings about something you have an emotional attachment to, which will help set you free.

The trick is to keep it to thirty minutes and tackle just one small area at a time, so the task doesn't feel overwhelming and risk draining your motivation rather than boosting it. How about taking on one of the following:

- **Your wardrobe.** Is it full of clothes you've forgotten you ever bought (and maybe wish you hadn't)? Choose a drawer or a section of your wardrobe and have a clear-out. Recycling what you don't need is good for your headspace, and good for the planet. Giving stuff away can release endorphins – those happy chemicals in the brain – as well as reducing waste, so consider charity shops or freecycling so someone else can make use of what you no longer need.
- **Your bedroom.** This is a sacred space, and clearing it of clutter allows energy to move and circulate freely. This will help you to get a deeper, more restful sleep.
- **The freezer.** Great for making space for some boxes of frozen banana, berries and mango, so you're ready to create any of my super smoothies (see pp. 69, 70 and 116).
- **Your kitchen cupboards.** Removing all the sugary snacks and junk that you don't want in your life anymore will create space for new, healthier foods, and take away temptation.

Reach out and connect

As human beings, we are wired to be social; we have a basic need to belong to a 'tribe'. In the past, as we evolved, we would have hunted, travelled and lived in tight social groups, and relied on one another for survival. But as time has gone on, our world has become more solitary. We are far more likely to be found head down, staring at our phone or laptop, buried in tasks, busy with 'stuff'. It's easy to get so consumed by our day-to-day lives that we forget to connect with the people we love and care about. But friendships are like plants; they don't thrive without care.

A few times a week, I try to reach out to a friend with a phone call, or maybe meet them for breakfast, head out for a walk together, grab a coffee or get in some training. Perhaps you've noticed a certain friend who might really need that connection right now – or maybe you're the one who needs a friendly ear. Either way, harnessing the power of connection can be incredibly beneficial for both you and them, physically and mentally.

Think of it as an energy exchange: when people are paying attention to each other, it can deepen the relationship, feel inspiring and build trust. There's scientific evidence that people with good friends and strong relationships who feel part of their community have lower stress levels, lower blood pressure and stronger immune systems and will live longer, healthier lives.

I was never someone who felt comfortable reaching out and sharing my feelings, especially as it involved appearing a little bit vulnerable. As a rugby player, there was definitely a feeling that you just had to 'man up'. Unfortunately, in the world we're in, and especially in macho, ego-fuelled sports like rugby, it's often seen as a weakness to show emotion. But as I've got older – and I like to think a little bit wiser – I have realized the power in reaching out and sharing, and not bottling up negative feelings or worries.

So, when you're feeling a bit overwhelmed or anxious, or like you're alone in the world, take a breath and make the decision to reach out to a friend. It could make all the difference to you both.

I really feel it's part of our nature as humans to connect with others and form relationships and bonds. So invest in a good social network – whether that's gym friends, school-gate friends, sports friends or neighbours. Make sure you meet up in real life, not just on WhatsApp or social media.

And why not extend your 'reaching out' practice to include talking to strangers? Make eye contact, smile, strike up conversations in the café or supermarket, and ask how people are doing. You'll be amazed at the response you get – and how good it makes you feel.

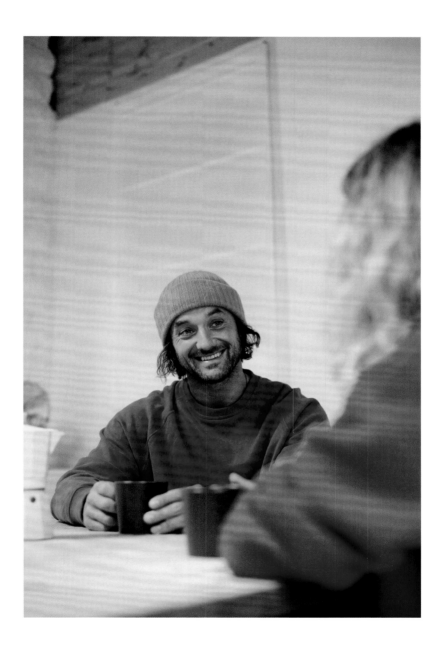

"

Imagine if you left it too late to do those things in life that you'd always wanted to do. Waited longer than you needed to make that leap into a life that felt right.

Don't keep putting it off. Today is always a good day to start fresh: make that choice, take the next step and follow your gut instinct.

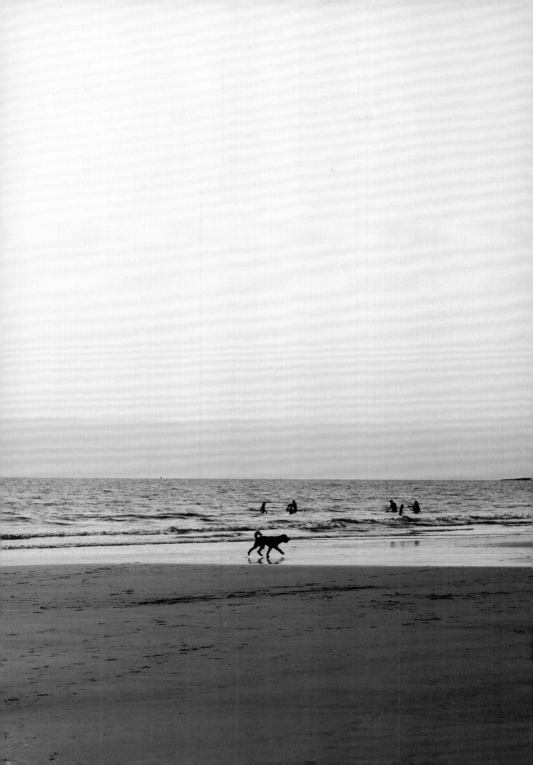

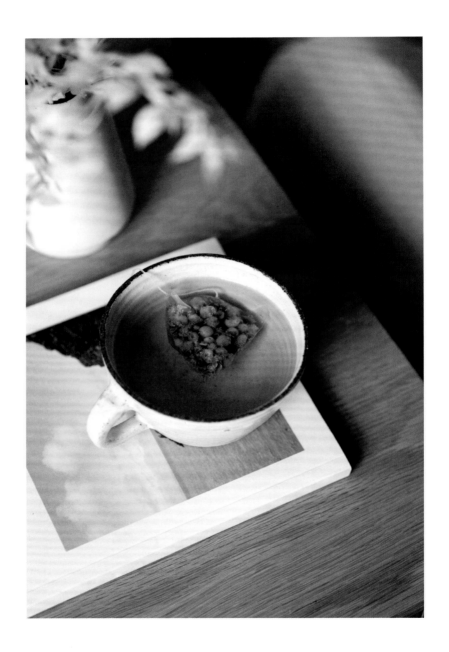

My ultimate bedtime routine

What's happened to our sleep? Research has shown that just in the past 70 years, we've lopped 20 per cent off our nightly sleep. What used to be 8 hours is now down to 6.8 hours – and it's falling further as we fragment our nights with caffeine, technology and hyperstimulated minds. Poor sleep is linked to everything from obesity and type 2 diabetes to heart disease and even Alzheimer's. So it's about time we all put sleep at the top of our list of priorities.

Here's my solution. You probably remember having a bedtime routine as a small child. Maybe it went something like this: bath, milk, story, then tucked into bed. But adults can benefit just as much from having a set of familiar pre-bed rituals. This routine gives the brain its cue that it's time to prepare for sleep, which means you will fall asleep more quickly and hopefully enjoy a deeper, more restful slumber.

Everyone will have a slightly different pattern that works for them, so experiment and see which rituals are most effective for you. However, these two are super-important:

- **Try to go to bed and wake up** at approximately the same time every day, even at weekends, if you can. Irregular sleep patterns mess with our circadian rhythm – the delicate internal clock that governs everything from our heart health to our weight and risk of disease. Lie-ins give you a kind of jet lag, so it's best to keep them to a maximum of one hour, as a rule.
- **Put away your phone,** laptop and tablet at least one hour before bed. That's important for two reasons. One is that screen time stimulates the brain and gives it a dopamine rush when it should be calming down and preparing for sleep. The other is that the blue light emitted by screens suppresses the body's production of the sleep hormone melatonin, so it kills your desire for shut-eye.

I have developed a bedtime routine based on the latest research, and I have to say it has helped me transform a very disrupted sleep cycle into a more consistently restorative one. If I don't sleep well one night, I can pretty much always trace it back to not committing enough time and effort to my usual pre-sleep rituals.

So, in addition to the two points above, here's what my routine involves:

- **No caffeine after midday.** Most people know not to drink coffee or caffeinated drinks in the evening, but caffeine lingers longer in the body than we think. Even six hours before bed, it can reduce sleep by up to an hour. I know if I drink coffee in the afternoon, my brain will be in overdrive that night.
- **Eat early in the evening.** It takes about two to three hours to digest a meal, and if your digestive system is working overtime, your body won't be able to sleep. I generally don't eat after 6 p.m., which gives my system plenty of time for digestion.

And thirty minutes before bed, this is what I do:

- **A mind dump.** Write down your to-do list for tomorrow, so you are offloading the contents of your mind. Keep a notepad by the bed if you need to, so you aren't tempted to use your phone for this. I do this as part of my five-minute journaling practice, which is a brilliant way of clearing the mind before sleep (see p. 108).
- **A calming drink.** I usually go for a camomile-based tea.
- **A hot bath.** I'll skip this on really busy days, but if I do have time for it, I seem to sleep deeper and wake up more refreshed. I add a muscle soak to the water (usually magnesium flakes) plus some lavender oil, and light some candles to set a good, calming vibe. I either read in the bath or listen to a sleep story on the Calm app.

- **Mood lighting.** I turn down all the dimmable lights in the house, and turn off the harshest lights. I also have an orange Himalayan salt lamp in my bedroom, which I find incredibly calming.
- **A bedtime flow.** Some gentle movement will release the tension of the day and relax tired muscles. I usually use the five-minute wind-down flow (see p. 92), or the fifteen-minute ultimate bedtime flow (see p. 146) if I have time.
- **A breath practice.** I use the five-minute wind-down breath practice (see p. 78). The key with wind-down breathwork is to inhale, hold your breath for the same count, then make the exhalation longer. This triggers the body's relaxation response. A breath practice is a kind of meditation, and research shows it can halve the time it takes for you to fall asleep.

I know that if I've done everything on my list, I'm off to the land of Nod in a couple of minutes and I'll wake up refreshed and ready to tackle another day. Happy sleeping!

Avocado and sweet potato buddha bowl

BREAKFAST   Serves 2

I found the Buddha bowl when I first visited Bali ten years ago, and I've been creating my own versions ever since. This one combines my love of colourful food with a variety of tasty, nutrient-packed goodies, to fill you up without putting you into a food coma.

200g sweet potato, peeled and diced
½ red onion, diced
1 tbsp extra-virgin olive oil
¼ tsp sweet smoked paprika
1 sprig rosemary, finely chopped
75g tenderstem broccoli, trimmed
2 large free-range eggs
250g pouch cooked glorious grains (or your choice of mixed grains, quinoa or beans)
2 handfuls baby spinach
100g cherry tomatoes, halved
2 sprigs basil leaves
½ large ripe avocado (stone removed), sliced
1 large handful alfalfa sprouts (see p. 264)
2 tbsp savoury seeds, toasted (see p. 265)

Preheat the oven to 200°C/180°C fan/Gas Mark 4.

Lay the sweet potato and onion on a lined oven tray. Pour the olive oil over the top and sprinkle with sweet paprika and rosemary. Season well with salt and pepper and mix until everything is well coated. Put into the oven for 15 minutes.

Remove the tray from the oven and add the broccoli, mixing it into the sweet potato and red onion, and then return to the oven for a further 10 minutes.

Meanwhile, bring a saucepan of water to the boil. When it is boiling, add the eggs and cook for 5–6 minutes. (This is if you like your yolks runny, if you like it firmer just cook it for 1–2 minutes longer.) While the eggs are cooking, heat up the grains.

When the eggs are cooked, remove from hot water and place into a bowl of cold water, to stop the cooking process and cool the eggs slightly. Peel and cut each one in half.

Divide the warm grains between two serving bowls. Remove the vegetables from the oven and add to the bowls, along with the spinach. Mix in the tomatoes with the basil leaves and season with salt and pepper. Add the avocado, alfalfa and eggs, sprinkle the seeds over the top and tuck in!

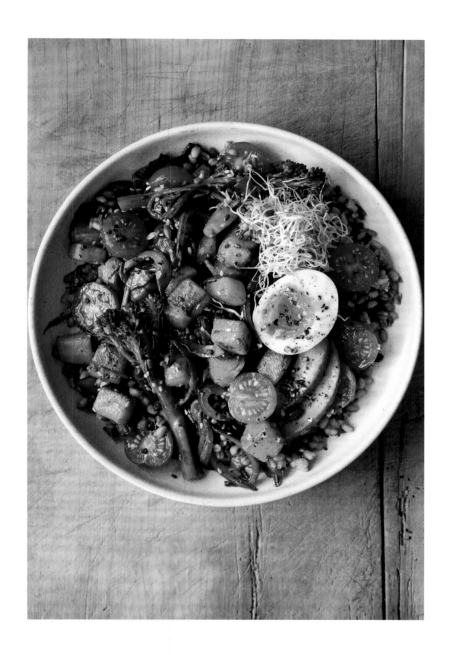

Homemade granola

I'm pretty sure I'm addicted to granola. I love that you can create something so simple with all your favourite crunchy and chewy things, and then add it to porridge, cereals or salads – or just smash it on its own, maybe with a little oat milk and honey.

300g jumbo rolled oats
150g mixed seeds (sunflower, sesame and pumpkin)
100g pecans, roughly chopped
75g flaked almonds
100ml coconut oil
150ml maple syrup
1 tsp vanilla extract
1 tsp ground cinnamon
½ tsp ground cardamom
½ tsp mixed spice
zest of 1 orange
1 tsp flaky sea salt
50g coconut flakes
150g mixed dried fruit, roughly chopped (cranberries, raisins, apricots, figs)
50g unsweetened banana chips
25g puffed spelt/wheat

Preheat the oven to 170°C/150°C fan/Gas Mark 3, and line two large trays with greaseproof paper.

Add the rolled oats, mixed seeds, pecans and almonds to a large bowl.

Put the coconut oil, maple syrup, vanilla extract, spices, orange zest and salt into a small saucepan and place over a medium heat. Stir well until the coconut oil has melted completely. Pour this over the oat mixture, and combine until well coated.

Divide the mixture between the two lined trays and spread out evenly. Put in the oven for 10 minutes.

Take the trays out of the oven and, using a wooden spoon, give the contents of each tray a good mix. Return them to the oven for a further 10 minutes.

Remove from the oven and sprinkle with the coconut flakes and dried fruit. Give both trays a good mix again and cook for another 10–15 minutes, or until the oats are a lovely nutty-brown colour.

Remove the trays from the oven and leave to cool. After about 10 minutes, add the banana chips and puffed wheat and mix one more time.

When completely cool, store in an airtight jar or container.

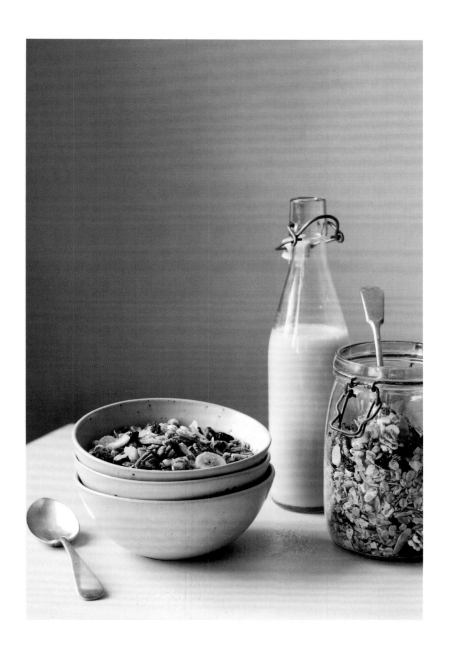

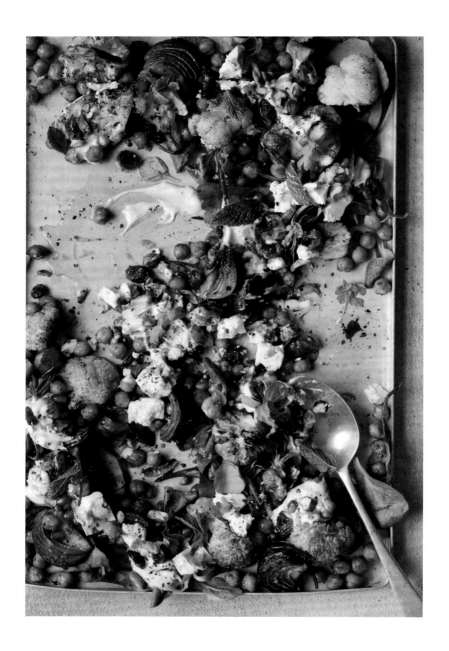

Roasted cauliflower and chickpea salad

LUNCH   Serves 4

Another meal that's come out of my leftover roast experiments, with flavours inspired by a dish I tried in the Philippines. I stumbled across a food stall down a little side street where they were roasting cauliflower and corn – and they had a big bowl of local greens to add to each plate. It was so simple and light and super-tasty – I've been trying to recreate it ever since.

1 large cauliflower, broken into florets
2 red onions, cut into wedges
2 x 400g cans chickpeas, drained
1 heaped tbsp ras el hanout
3 tbsp extra-virgin olive oil
1 large handful mint leaves, roughly chopped
2 large handfuls coriander, roughly chopped
100g mixed salad leaves
3 tbsp dried cranberries, roughly chopped
50g feta cheese, crumbled
2 tbsp pomegranate molasses (optional)
30g pistachios, roughly chopped
50g pomegranate seeds

Dressing
150ml natural yoghurt
2 tbsp tahini
juice of ½ lemon
3 tbsp water

Preheat the oven to 200°C/180°C fan/Gas Mark 6, and line two large trays with greaseproof paper.

Put the cauliflower, red onion, chickpeas, ras el hanout and olive oil into a large bowl. Season well with salt and pepper, and mix until everything has a good coating of oil and spice. Divide between the two trays, and spread out as a single layer on each. Roast for 25–30 minutes, making sure to turn the cauliflower halfway through.

Meanwhile, whisk the dressing ingredients together.

Remove the mixture from the oven, add the mint and coriander and stir well. Divide the salad leaves between two bowls and spoon the dressing over the leaves. Top with the cauliflower and chickpea mixture.

Sprinkle the cranberries and feta cheese on top, and drizzle with the pomegranate molasses (if using). Lastly, sprinkle with the pistachios and pomegranate seeds.

Roasted squash and aubergine noodle bowl

LUNCH   Serves 4

Noodles are super-fast to make but not always that exciting, so I find adding squash and a little extra heat to this recipe makes it the perfect lunch to fire me up for the rest of the day. You'll often find roasted veg in my creations, as they're an easy way to add colour, flavour and texture to any dish.

500g butternut squash, peeled
    and cut into wedges
2 small aubergines, each cut into
    8 wedges
1 heaped tsp mild curry powder
2 tbsp mild olive oil
200g rice noodles
1 large handful coriander,
    roughly chopped
    including stems
½ large cucumber, julienned
1 large carrot, peeled and
    julienned
6 radishes, thinly sliced
2 handfuls beansprouts
2 spring onions, finely sliced
40g peanuts, roughly chopped
4 tbsp savoury seeds, toasted
    (see p. 265)

Dressing
30g palm sugar, finely chopped
2 tbsp boiling water
2 long red chillies, deseeded
    and finely diced
juice of 1 lime
2 tbsp rice vinegar
2 tbsp light soy sauce

Preheat the oven to 220°C/200°C fan/Gas Mark 7.

Line two large trays with greaseproof paper. Place the butternut squash and aubergine onto the two trays. Sprinkle with curry powder and a little salt and pepper. Drizzle with the oil, and mix so everything is well coated. Put into the oven for 20 minutes.

Meanwhile, place the noodles into a large heatproof bowl and pour boiling water over them until they are covered. Leave them until they have softened.

Next make the dressing. Put the palm sugar and boiling water into a small bowl and mix until the sugar has dissolved completely. Add the remaining ingredients and stir well.

Drain the noodles and return them to the heatproof bowl. Add half of the dressing to the noodles, along with the chopped coriander, and mix well.

Divide the noodles among four serving bowls. Add the cucumber, carrot, radishes and beansprouts to each bowl. Remove the roasted veg from the oven and divide between the four bowls. Top with spring onions, peanuts, seeds and the remaining dressing.

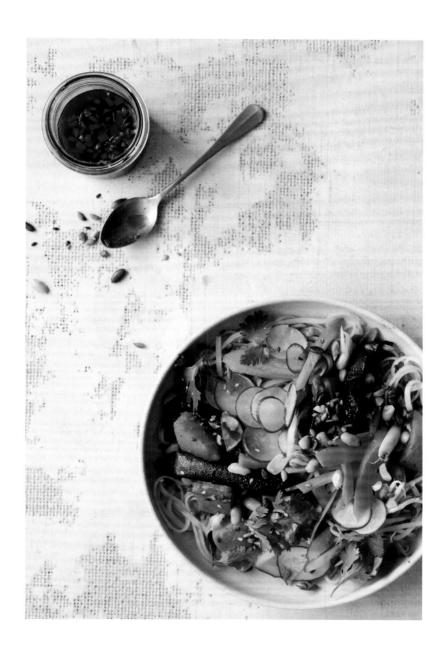

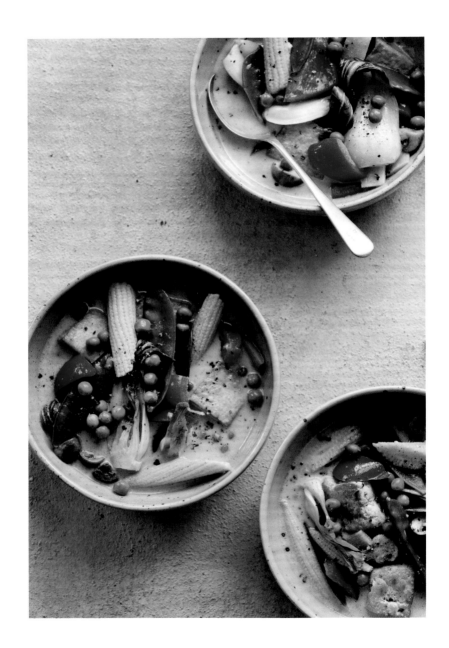

Veggie combo coconut curry

DINNER

Serves 2

As a kid I lived in the Middle East, and I remember most of our meals involved curry, so it has become a crucial dish in my diet. Over the years I've tried the local cuisine and all sorts of curry creations while exploring different countries, and this combo has become my go-to weeknight dish to satisfy a curry craving.

1 tbsp vegetable oil
250g firm tofu, cut into cubes
1½ tbsp Thai green curry paste
    (I use Mae Ploy)
300ml vegetable stock
400ml coconut milk
2 kaffir lime leaves (see p. 265)
100g button mushrooms
75g baby corn
120g bamboo shoots
1 red pepper, cut into
    2.5-cm chunks
75g mangetout
1 tsp palm sugar, finely chopped
2 tsp light soy sauce
3 baby pak choi, trimmed,
    leaves separated
50g frozen peas

Place a medium non-stick sauté pan or wok over a high heat. When smoking hot, add the oil and tofu and cook until the tofu has browned lightly on all sides.

Next, add the curry paste and stir well for 1 minute. Then add the stock and half of the coconut milk and the lime leaves. Bring up to a simmer and add the mushrooms, corn and bamboo shoots, and cook for 3 minutes before adding the pepper. Cook for 1 minute more and then add the remaining coconut milk, as well as the mangetout, palm sugar and soy sauce.

Cook for a further minute before adding the pak choi and peas. Once the pak choi has wilted, remove from heat and serve immediately.

Ginger fire shot

I have my mate Marcus in Sweden to thank for this spicy fire starter. We made a big batch of it to kick-start every morning before training; it blew my mind then and it still does to this day!

300g ginger
½ long red chilli, sliced
    (or one whole chilli if
    you like it really spicy)
80g honey
juice of 3 lemons

Grate the ginger directly into a medium saucepan – that way you don't lose any of its precious juice. There's no need to peel it, just grate it all up, skin and all.

Pour 1.5 litres of water into the pan and add the chilli. Put over a low-medium heat and bring up to a gentle simmer. This should take about 10 minutes.

Lower the heat and continue to cook gently for another 10 minutes. Leave to cool slightly, then drain the liquid through a sieve and mix in the honey. Once completely cool, stir in the lemon juice. Pour into sterilized bottles and keep in the fridge. This mixture makes a big batch, but it will last in the fridge for 5–7 days.

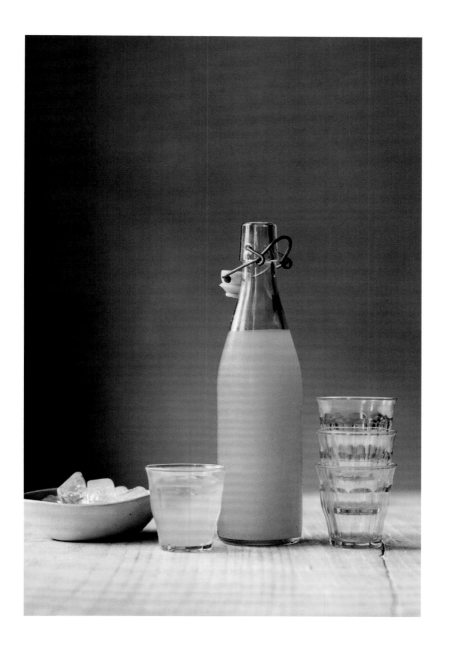

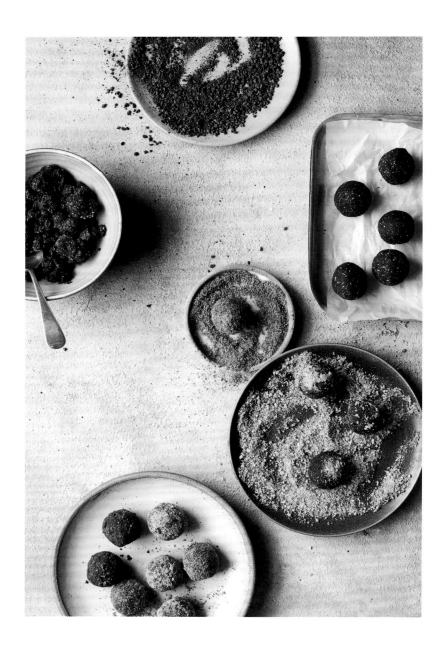

Supercharged power balls

Makes 20 balls

I first had one of these at an organic farmers' market in Australia; they were handing out samples with a coffee . . . I think I then hung around for an hour, slowly devouring the rest of the plate. We became good friends for life (me and the balls).

200g Medjool dates, chopped
100ml boiling water
150g rolled oats
50g pumpkin seeds
50g sunflower seeds
50g flaked almonds, toasted
3 tbsp chia seeds
80g cocoa powder
80g peanut butter
1 tsp vanilla extract
2 tbsp honey
large pinch sea salt

To coat
30g pistachios, ground to
    a powder
30g milled flaxseed
20g cacao nibs

Put the dates in small heatproof bowl. Pour the boiling water in and cover the bowl with cling film. Leave for 10–15 minutes.

Meanwhile, put the oats, pumpkin and sunflower seeds, almonds, chia seeds, cocoa powder, peanut butter, vanilla, honey and sea salt into a food processor.

Add the dates and water, and pulse the mixture until combined. If it sticks to the sides of the food processor, remove the lid and push the mixture down with a rubber spatula before continuing to pulse.

Next, divide the mixture into 20 evenly sized balls. Roll each ball in the palm of your hand to shape it.

Place the pistachios, flaxseed and cacao nibs into three small bowls (one ingredient per bowl). Roll each ball into one of the coatings and place on a tray. Pop into the fridge until needed.

Raw carrot-cake balls

SNACKS Makes 20 balls

I'm in a similar love affair with these. I wanted to get creative with the ingredients and look at healthier and quirkier flavour combos, and now I have a ball recipe for all occasions! These make a great snack to travel with, so I can get a burst of energy wherever I happen to be.

100g Medjool dates, chopped
100g dried apricots, diced
100ml boiling water
100g walnuts, toasted
100g rolled oats
200g grated carrot
50g desiccated coconut
3 tbsp milled flaxseed
zest of ½ orange
1 tsp vanilla extract
1 tsp ground cinnamon
1 tsp mixed spice

To coat
50g desiccated coconut

Put the dates and apricots into a small heatproof bowl. Pour the boiling water on top and cover the bowl with cling film. Leave for 10–15 minutes.

Meanwhile, put the walnuts, oats, carrot, coconut, milled flaxseed, orange zest, vanilla, cinnamon and mixed spice into a food processor.

Making sure to keep the soaking water afterwards, drain the dried fruit through a sieve. Add the fruit to the food processor and pulse until everything is combined. If the mixture is a little dry, add a little of the soaking liquid and pulse again.

Divide the mixture into 20 evenly sized balls. Roll each ball in the palm of your hand to shape it, then roll each ball in desiccated coconut to coat. Put in the fridge to keep for snack time, or they will keep in a sealed container somewhere cool.

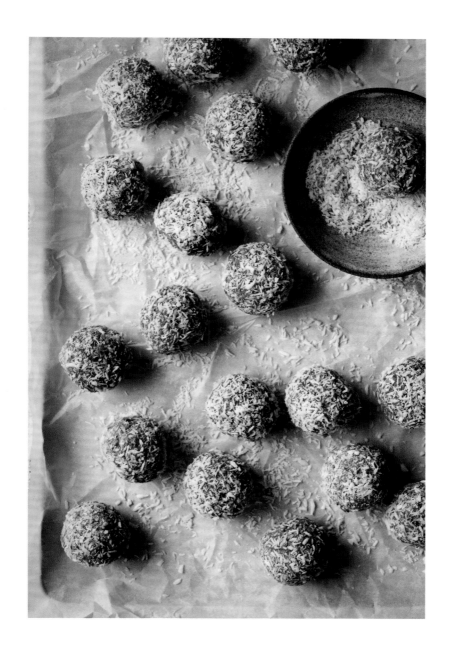

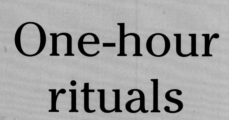

One-hour
rituals

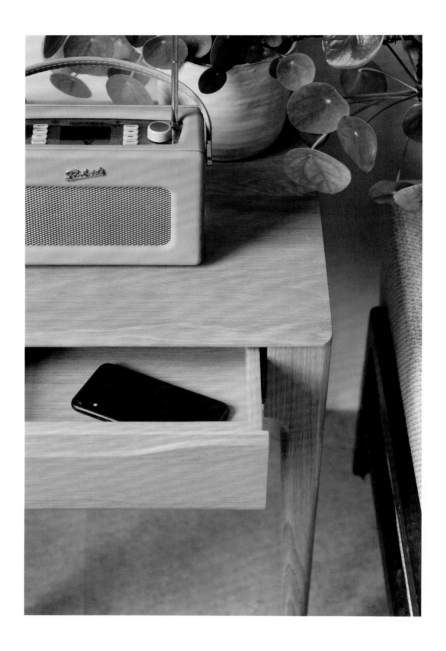

The five-step tech zombie hack

Unless you plan to become a goat herder or a hermit, we have to accept that our phones aren't going anywhere. Our world is only becoming more digital, so for me it's about finding healthier ways to manage technology. But it's really important that we do, because we are not robots, we're humans – and humans need connection, sunlight, communication and movement. Human beings probably don't need to be swiping and tapping their phone 2,617 times a day, as one study estimated (rising to 5,427 times for the top 10 per cent of users).

Science shows we are being pulled into these vortexes of technology; every time we swipe we get a little shot of the pleasure hormone dopamine. It doesn't take long before our brain becomes hooked and we're constantly searching for that little high – and we lose control.

That's why I want you to commit an hour to planning how to take five steps towards restoring balance when it comes to tech.

First, have a look at your phone's screen time log, to find out how many hours a week you use it, what apps you're using most, and the time of day you're using them. Write down your 'weak' areas, then list the five steps you're going to take that will allow you more headspace and freedom away from your phone.

These are the five steps I have taken with my own tech use, and ones I recommend:

1. **No-tech mornings.** Keep the first 30 minutes of your day phone-free, which means not keeping it by your bed and using it as an alarm clock. Buy an alarm clock! When your phone is the first thing you touch before you even get out of bed, it sets you on that feedback loop of endless checking and scrolling, and can mean you start the day on a negative and stressful note. So focus instead on building a morning routine that's dedicated to looking

after yourself. Do a breathing exercise and a movement flow and make a healthy breakfast before you allow yourself online.

2. **Phone-free lunches.** Keep your phone away from the table (or wherever you're eating). That way, you will eat more slowly and mindfully, and are less likely to overeat. It also gives you a mini phone detox, so you can gather your thoughts and focus your energy on getting through the rest of the working day.

3. **Use tech to manage tech.** Use your phone's features to monitor your use, set limits on the apps you tend to overuse, and set daily screen-time limits. This will help you build boundaries into your day. Consider 'hiding' some tempting apps in a folder on your home screen, which can help you to avoid that zombie 'pick up phone, check Instagram' urge.

4. **Turn off notifications.** Just seeing or hearing those bleeps and pings is enough to distract you, even if you decide not to act on them. I set my notifications each morning, depending on what's urgent that day. Generally, though, I have them turned off.

5. **Dial back with 'do not disturb'.** Use your phone's 'do not disturb' feature when you really want to get something done. This will silence all notifications, including phone calls, for as long as it is enabled. I have found this is a great way to find some focus and clarity.

Random acts of kindness

Doing something for someone else without expecting anything in return can light up their life, but it can also bring a warm glow to your own.

Being kind is a superpower that results in all kinds of mental and physical payback. It's so easy to go through life on autopilot, being busy in your own world and not looking up to notice other people or their needs. We can all feel a bit disconnected at times, which makes us lonely.

I find that just smiling at strangers in the street and keeping an eye out for people who might need your help can lift your mood. Maybe you could carry someone's bag if they look like they need help? Or chat with someone who looks lonely?

It can be even more impactful to set aside an hour in your day to look for opportunities to perform a random act of kindness – stepping out of your little bubble to shine a light in someone else's life. By doing that, you will make them feel like they matter. And in return, you feel like you're worth something too. It doesn't have to be a grand gesture, it's more about little choices and simple interactions.

Here are some ideas:

- **Bake a cake or cook a meal,** and take it round to someone you know is having a hard time right now.
- **Wrap tiny presents** and leave them, along with a note, in random places like your local café.
- **Bring a small bunch of flowers** to someone you don't often acknowledge, like the doctor's receptionist or a corner shop owner.
- **Offer to do the shopping** for an elderly neighbour or someone with a new baby, or perhaps you could walk their dog.
- **Send a letter to a grandparent,** parent or someone else you haven't seen in a while.

The effects of kindness on your body are quite startling. According to the science, helping others can:

- **Generate the hormone oxytocin,** which promotes feelings of love, trust and well-being.
- **Protect the heart.** Oxytocin causes the release of nitric oxide in the body, which expands the blood vessels and lowers blood pressure.
- **Stimulate the part** of the nervous system that triggers the body's relaxation response.
- **Reduce stress.** People who help or volunteer tend to have less of the stress hormone cortisol in their bodies.
- **Give you what's known as a 'helper's high',** where natural opiates and the reward chemical dopamine are released from the brain.
- **Lift your mood.** One study showed that people who engaged in random acts of kindness were more likely to feel a boost in mood than those who gave themselves little treats.

So why not try this experiment . . . Pledge to be kind to a stranger every day for a week: offer to carry shopping, pay people compliments, and reach out to people in need. Keep a note of your feelings after each act: how has it changed your mindset?

Blue power-up

To me, there's nothing quite like being in the open water to make me feel alive, invigorated and utterly liberated. Nothing beats that sensation, and I would love for you to spend an hour in the ocean or swimming in a local pond or lake so you can tap into the incredible health benefits too.

Discovering surfing was a key tool in healing my body and mind. I didn't know it then, but ocean and surf therapy are well-recognized treatments for anxiety and mental health problems, and this is all backed up by scientific research.

I think the power of being in open water lies in the fact that it works on so many physical and mental levels. First of all, you are outside, with no access to your phone and no tech, completely at one with nature. That feeling of being utterly disconnected is truly liberating, and that's not really possible anywhere on land now. Then there's the emotional release you get from being in cold water. It's hard to explain, and it's a slightly different experience for everyone – I have seen people giggle uncontrollably, for example. But for me it's about having the freedom to move unrestricted, the awe I feel at Mother Nature, and the reaction of my body to the cold water.

Research shows that when we immerse our bodies in cold water, our brains release huge amounts of feel-good chemicals, like dopamine, which improve your mood and give you a boost of positive energy.

In the first few moments after entering the water, your body will probably be shouting at you to get out. Fear sets in and your heart rate spikes, and this is when you need to call on your breath – just as we talked about in the section on taking a cold shower (see p. 143). Inhale slowly, deeply and steadily, and lengthen your exhale to promote feelings of calm.

I find that it is when I step out of my body's instinctive response to panic that I feel most alive and invigorated. It is as if the shock is a wake-up to your system: it forces you to feel fully present and focused. There can be literally nothing else on your mind. That's why I think being in open water is the quickest and most effective form of mindfulness ever.

When you are surfing, you add in an extra bit of fear and awe, and it is leaning into that fear that improves your resilience to stress. I've certainly found it translates into other areas of my life, so it's no surprise that research has shown that a 30-minute surfing session can improve your mood – and surfing is being used more and more in mental health initiatives.

Wild swimming in lakes, ponds and rivers can also unlock incredible benefits for both the body and the mind. It has a natural meditative effect: you're totally in the moment, focusing on your breathing, timing and technique, and the slow, steady rhythm of swimming steadies the nervous system and promotes relaxation.

Swimming is also great exercise if you are looking to build up a greater range of motion. It is low-impact because of the weightlessness you feel, it is easy on your joints, improves flexibility and core strength, and it is also a total body workout. Find your nearest wild swimming spot at www.swimming.org/openwater or www.outdoorswimmingsociety.com.

So start making plans to head out into the open water – you won't regret it. And if you don't want to get in the water, you can still reap its benefits. Even staring at the ocean and hearing the waves ebb and flow can change the brain's frequency, relaxing us and putting us into a mild meditative state.

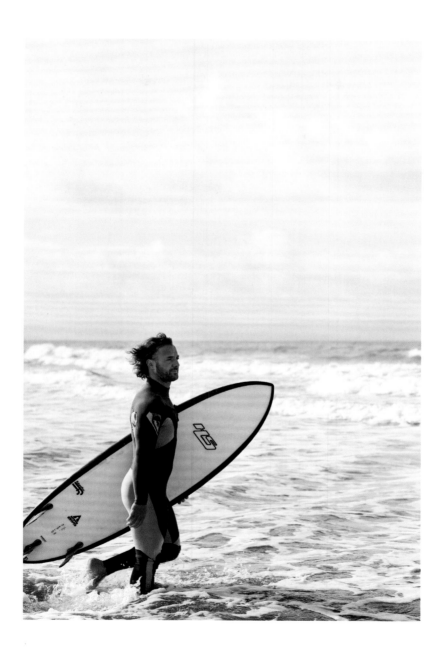

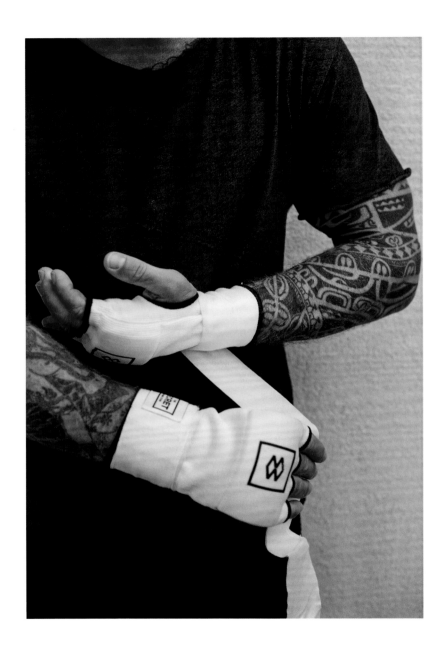

Commit to doing something new

Learning something new is like taking a powerful brain-stimulating drug. When you step out of your everyday autopilot mode and challenge yourself to try something you haven't done before, it actually physically changes the structure of your brain. Every time I think of that, it blows my mind just a little bit more.

Committing to new activities regularly has multiple benefits:

- **It generates new brain cells,** no matter what age you are, which can both combat and prevent depression – as well as help reduce anxiety.
- **It helps form new connections** between the brain cells, and new pathways within the brain.
- **It can help reduce** the risk of dementia in later life.
- **It produces the happy hormone** dopamine, and improves your mood and overall mental health.

Doing routine things doesn't have the same effect, because your body and brain become used to those activities and don't need to think too hard. Essentially, you get stuck in a rut. It's novelty that challenges the brain and keeps it healthy.

It's a similar story with the body: if you are continually moving it in the same way, it adapts to the stress you are putting on it and you will stop seeing progress in your fitness goals. You could also end up with overuse injuries.

Here are some ideas for new activities that will challenge your brain and body. Alternatively, if you have something on your to-do list that you have always wanted to try but never got around to, commit today to checking it out. You know what they say – use it or lose it!

- **Join a dance class.** All exercise releases endorphins, the brain's happy chemicals, but dancing releases even more. Dancing is a powerful mental health tool, and something none of us do enough!
- **Try boxing.** It torches calories, improves focus and relieves tension. It is also a workout for the brain because it is so strategic.
- **Start yoga,** if you haven't tried it before. Yoga relieves stress and helps you manage anxiety. Some forms of yoga seem to dampen the body's stress response, which can help your immune system function better. That might be why people who practise yoga regularly say that it helps autoimmune conditions like alopecia and lupus.
- **Have a surf lesson.** Surfing is a whole-body workout, improves balance and coordination, and is a brilliant concentration- and mood-booster.
- **Go back to a team sport.** Many of you won't have played on a team since school, so join one now to get active and make new friends. In addition to the general benefits of exercise, playing team sports improves self-esteem and increases life satisfaction.
- **Put a stargazing app on your phone,** and spend an hour finding constellations on the next clear night.
- **Join a local book or film club** – or start one.

The trick is to step out of your comfort zone just enough to be challenged, but not so much that you feel overwhelmed.

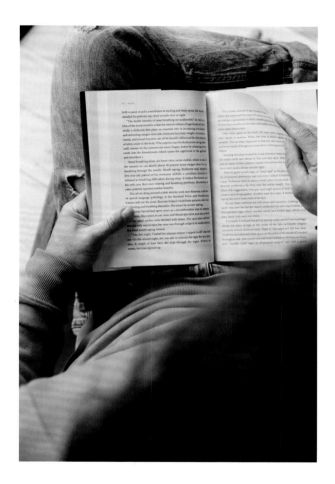

Listen to your emotions

P a u s e. Just because you're busy, it doesn't mean you're being productive. When your world gets a little busy and overwhelming, it tends to take over, right? Messing with the way you feel, think, react and behave? As that self-sabotage builds momentum, we often let it consume us, potentially leading to a whole chain of negativity.

I find that if you can pause when you recognize something is not 'feeling right' (even if you just take a few minutes), check in on how you're feeling, understand what energy is fuelling your emotions and take a few conscious breaths, everything becomes a little clearer and you can choose to change that vibration.

You can then go about your day a bit more mindfully, and not ninja-kick anyone in the face.

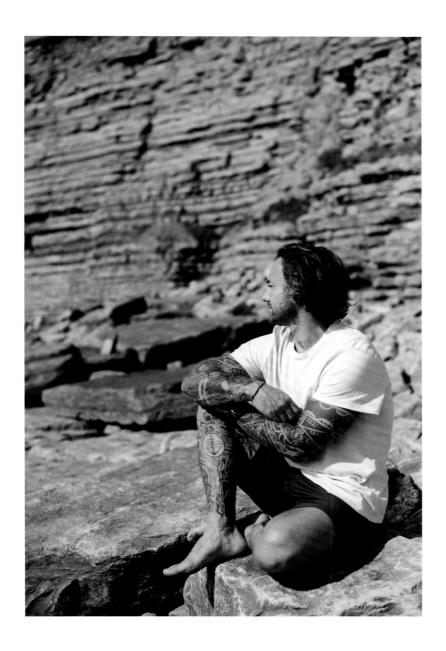

Veggie belly warmer

DINNER

Serves 4

This was a key part of my childhood when we were sick or needed a warm meal to cheer us up. Mum would use all the veggies in the fridge, and freestyle a little to make sure it was colourful and packed with plenty of nutrients. It was one of the first meals I made when I moved away from home, and it's still one of my top-ten recipes today.

650g butternut squash, cut into
   3-cm chunks
1 tbsp mild olive oil
2 tbsp ghee (or butter)
1 onion, thinly sliced
3 garlic cloves, finely chopped
5-cm piece of ginger, finely
   chopped
2 heaped tsp black/brown
   mustard seeds
2 heaped tsp cumin seeds
1 tsp ground turmeric
1 long red chilli, finely sliced
1 large handful curry leaves
350g red lentils
1 litre vegetable stock
400ml coconut milk
250g pouch cooked puy lentils
   (or a can of your favourite
   beans)
3 large handfuls baby spinach

Garnish
2 tomatoes, diced
1 long red chilli, finely sliced
handful fresh coriander, roughly
   chopped
handful roasted cashews,
   roughly chopped

To serve
toasted naan bread wedges

Preheat the oven to 200°C/180°C fan/Gas Mark 6, and line a large tray with greaseproof paper. Place the butternut squash onto the tray and drizzle with the olive oil. Season with salt and pepper and mix well. Put into the oven for 35 minutes.

Meanwhile, heat the ghee (or butter) in a large non-stick saucepan, add the onion and cook until it turns golden brown. Next add the garlic and ginger, and cook for 1 minute before adding the mustard seeds and cumin seeds. Stir well, and cook until the seeds begin to pop.

Add the turmeric, 1 red chilli and the curry leaves. Stir well for 1 minute and then add the red lentils and vegetable stock and bring up to a simmer. Cook with the lid on for 15 minutes, or until the lentils are tender.

Stir in the coconut milk and puy lentils (or beans), and bring back up to the simmer – then stir in the spinach and cook until it wilts. Pour in bowls, top with the garnishes that you like, and serve with toasted naan wedges for dipping!

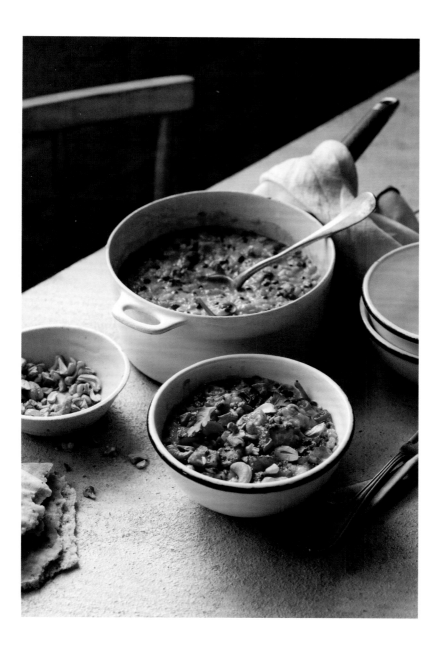

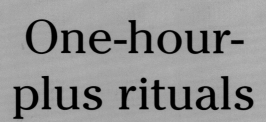

One-hour-plus rituals

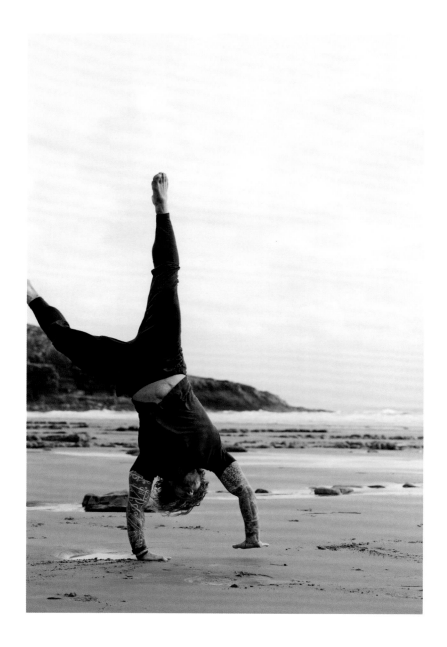

Play like a child

Playtime – it's my favourite time. Playing makes me happy, lifts my mood and keeps me active and feeling high on life. We should all do more of it, every single day. So why do we somehow feel guilty for making time to play? I think it's because society sees play as something children do. There's a feeling that, by the time we're adults, we should have grown out of such time-wasting silliness.

But that's not true. Just because we've grown up, our brains and bodies don't lose the need for novelty and the pleasure that play brings. As the playwright George Bernard Shaw once said: 'We don't stop playing because we grow old; we grow old because we stop playing.'

We complain that there is no time in our busy lives to play, but I think that's a lie we tell ourselves. We make time for everything else – work, chores, family, TV, endless phone scrolling. Hands up, you know it's true. What's more likely is that to clear time in a super-busy life for something so apparently random and indulgent as a few hours spent playing seems too difficult.

I am here to tell you that it isn't that difficult. In fact, it's really important to make time to play. Life is way too short for it to be Groundhog Day; we all deserve to have a little more of the fun stuff and a bit more passion and creative vibes flowing into our day.

Science is behind me on this one. Because playing absorbs and engages us fully, it gets our brains into what psychologists call a 'flow state'. That's when you feel so totally immersed in an activity that you lose track of time and have this feeling of utter focus and energy. Time spent in 'flow' makes us happy; it's calming and gives us clarity.

So it's no surprise that research shows that playful adults report a better sense of well-being, and they also live healthier, more active lives. They have lower levels of stress than more serious, less playful adults do. But here is the really interesting thing: in one study, playful people were shown to be able to develop coping strategies to deal with the stress in their lives, and were less likely to want to avoid or escape from potentially stressful and difficult situations.

Here are some tips for making play a priority in your life:

- **Give yourself permission to play every day.** Tell yourself it is therapy if you need to, but be sure to carve out little blocks of time for playing.
- **Think about what you loved doing as a child** and how you could recreate that today. Was it skateboarding you loved? Playing Lego? Drawing and colouring? Mountain biking?
- **Surround yourself with others who like to play.** Find out what your friends would secretly love to do and make plans right now!
- **Make time to play with the children in your life.** This can remind us of the magic of play, and hopefully rekindle something long-buried in our super-serious adult brains. Having my energetic godkids, nieces and nephews around me never fails to lift my mood, bring out the best in me and remind me of the importance of a playful and adventurous mind.

You have one life. Don't let it slip by, and don't waste it on the dull stuff.

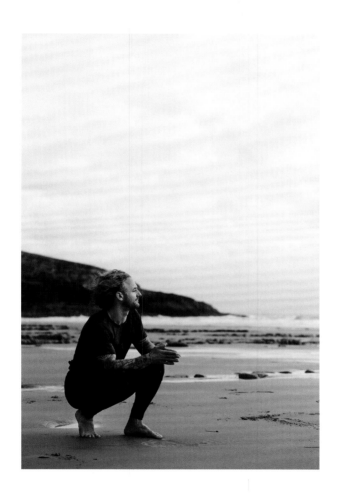

What is your priority?

Imagine if you found out that you only had a few more days left. You might glance back over your thoughts, fears and worries, and remember all the adventures you put off, all the choices you made because it was easier to just give in and give up. Maybe you've steered your life down a path that didn't feel right, but you did it because it's what someone else thought was right for you, or because you cared too much about other people's opinions and so you held back and played it safe.

The clock is ticking, the bus is rolling, and one day it's going to come to a stop. We all need reminding how fragile life can be, and how much more potential we all have to make our lives count and have an impact while we're here. Tap into your superpower and go share it with the world.

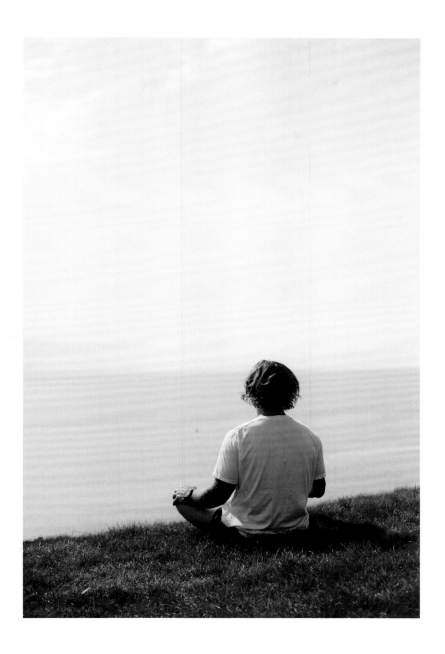

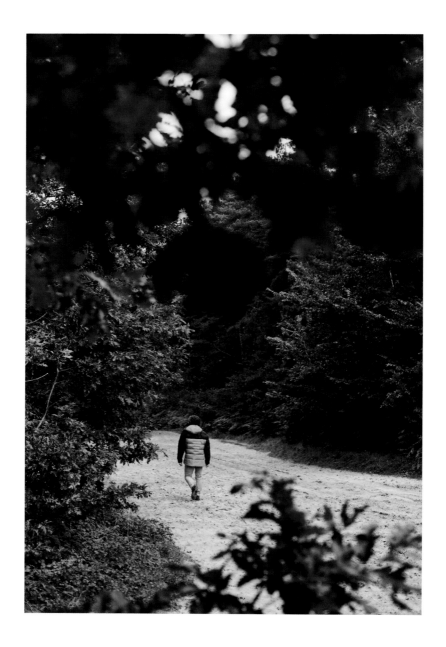

A deep dive into nature

Hopefully by now you have been so convinced by my passion and love for nature that you have made outdoor mini adventures part of your weekly routine (see p. 185).

Here is where we take it one step further. Any time we can spend in nature – even a few minutes – has real and proven benefits for our health. But when you can spend longer outside in green spaces, that's where magic happens.

There is something about immersing yourself deeply in nature for several hours – or even a full day – that provides incredible peace and calm.

A deep dive in nature is a powerful tool for our mental health. One study showed that people who went on a 90-minute walk in nature managed to break their negative thought loops. When their brains were scanned afterwards, they showed less neural activity in the area linked to the risk of mental illness than those who walked for exactly the same time but in an urban area.

We now know how long we should spend in nature every week to maximize all the health benefits: somewhere between two and five hours. That was based on a study of 20,000 people, so it's pretty solid evidence. But many of us are not managing anywhere near that. We are becoming a more inactive and deskbound species: it is estimated we spend about 90 per cent of our time indoors. And according to one survey, most adults have hardly – or never – listened to birdsong or smelled wild flowers in the past year.

Yet the evidence is clear from over 1,000 studies that immersing yourself in nature:

- **Lowers blood pressure.**
- **Cuts stress hormone levels.**
- **Improves self-esteem** and confidence.
- **Reduces anxiety.**
- **Lifts mood,** and gives a sense of meaning and purpose in life.

- **Sharpens memory** and hones concentration.
- **Boosts imagination** and creativity.

Here are some ideas for your deep dive into nature:

- **Have a picnic.** When was the last time you went out with your rug and a bag of food, and sat under a tree to eat? Rediscover life's simple pleasures – you won't regret it. (And if you have kids, they'll love it too.)
- **Explore a new green space.** Can you take the train or bus somewhere and navigate your way back without Google Maps? Can you find a cycle path or route you didn't know existed and spend a few hours pedalling?
- **Discover your local river or canal.** Is there a towpath you can walk along? Can you book a paddleboarding or kayaking session?
- **Walk in the woods.** Walking in the woods is proven to lower blood pressure and stress levels, and strengthens the immune system. The air in forests contains more oxygen, plus phytochemicals from natural tree oils. Phytochemicals are the scents you inhale in the woods, and they actually increase the number of 'killer cells' in your body which fight infection and boost your immune system.
- **Go to the beach.** When was the last time you dug a sandcastle, breathed in the sea air or jumped over waves?
- **Discover nature's larder.** Buy a guide to wild food, and set off on a foraging mission in a woodland or wild space near you. What you can find will depend on the season, but even if you only pick blackberries, it's a start.

So what are you waiting for? Rediscover that feeling of the breeze against your face, the sight of the sun's rays filtering through the leaves, and the sound of birdsong on a spring morning . . .

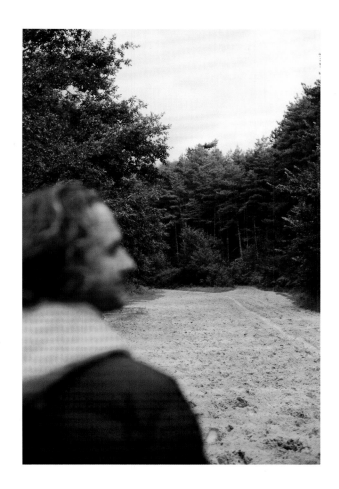

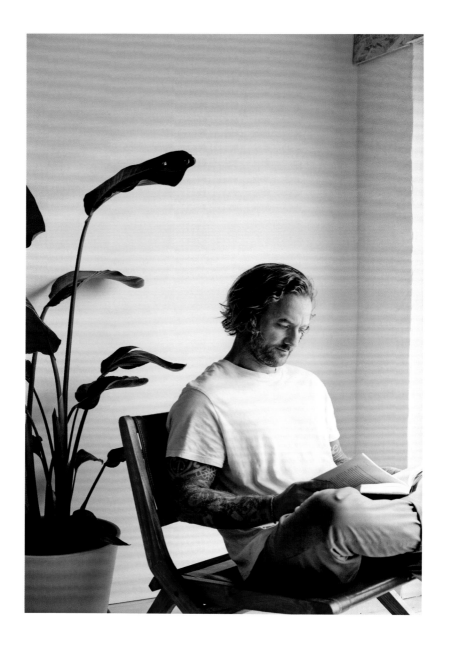

Digital detox

If you have already put into action the five-step tech zombie hack (see p. 219), you should notice you are becoming less reliant on your phone. But are you still getting the urge to pick it up less often for mindless scrolling?

You need to build in some times in the week where you don't have access to your phone at all. Why is this important? Science is beginning to discover that having your phone near you is a massive distraction, even when it's switched off. It saps your concentration so much that it actually drains your brain and reduces cognitive capacity.

Our ultimate aim should be to spend a few hours each week completely away from our phones. You can start by leaving it at home when you walk to the shops or pop out for 15 minutes. It might feel strange at first, as if you've forgotten something really important. The first time I did this, I kept patting my pocket instinctively and I felt a bit anxious.

It gets easier with time, and once you have mastered short trips out, progress to longer periods without your phone – like going out for meals or for a workout. It doesn't count if you turn it to airplane mode or switch it off; you actually have to leave it at home. This exercises your 'digital detox muscle' and prepares you for even longer times spent phone-free.

How you manage this is up to you and the patterns of your life. I have friends and clients who aim for a 5:2 or 12:2 phone diet – a phone fast for two days (or two part-days) per week or fortnight. That might mean one weekend day without your phone and one weekday evening where you don't use it at all.

I find that two half-days at the weekend with no access to my phone works perfectly to clear my mind and reset my tech boundaries. The real beauty is in what you choose to do instead – something deeply and richly rewarding, rather than a quick dopamine hit.

Here are some ideas:

- **Get outside for a deep dive into nature** (see p. 243) or a wild swim (see p. 223).
- **Sit down and read a whole book,** something you might not have done for years.
- **Plant something in the garden** or some herbs in a window box, or tackle a job in the house you've been putting off for ages.
- **Get some friends round** to watch a movie from beginning to end with no distractions, and chat about it afterwards.
- **Spend time with your family:** play board games, chat, go for a run or walk together. Really connect.
- **Sit in a green space** and observe nature around you; drink in the sights, sounds and smells. Observe the seasonal cues. Lie on your back and cloud-spot.
- **Spend time in the kitchen** doing something that will really absorb you: making fresh pasta or baking bread, for example.
- **Go outside and paint or draw.** Or sew/craft something at home, or do some mindful colouring.

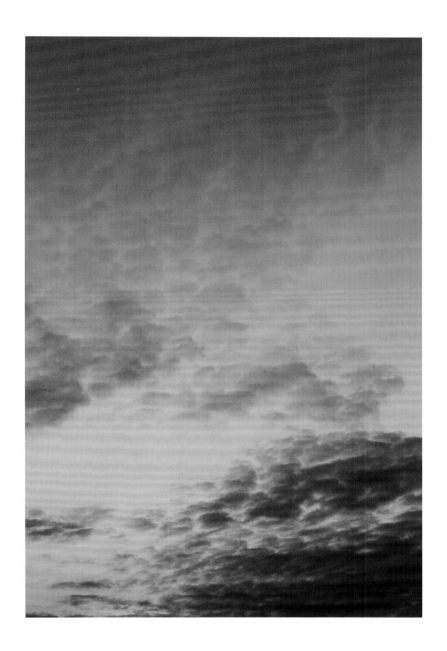

Take a breather

Find calm amongst the noise. No matter how busy you are, or that you think you're achieving your best and being your most productive, if you push through the signs your body gives you to stop and rest, you will suffer from stress (and not the good kind). And if stress is not managed, it becomes toxic and messes up those physical and mental signals.

The good news is that this can be prevented. You don't have to sacrifice lots of your precious time to be rewarded with more energy, a focused mind, better vibes and a big fat smile (win). Just find a few moments to pause, switch off – ideally closing your eyes – and:

- Inhale for five seconds
- Pause for a second
- Exhale for five seconds

That's it. The power of breath.
Now let's get to it.

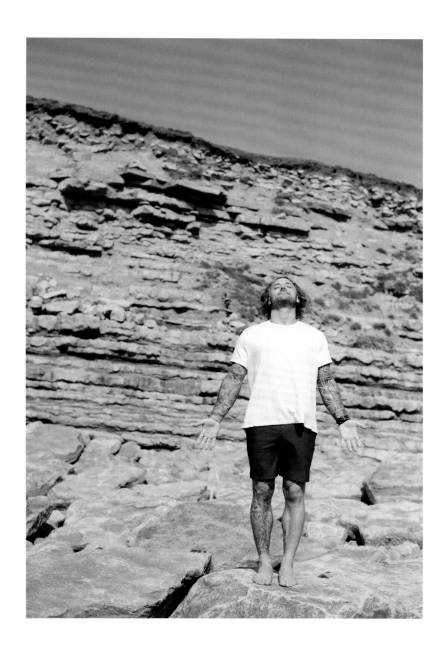

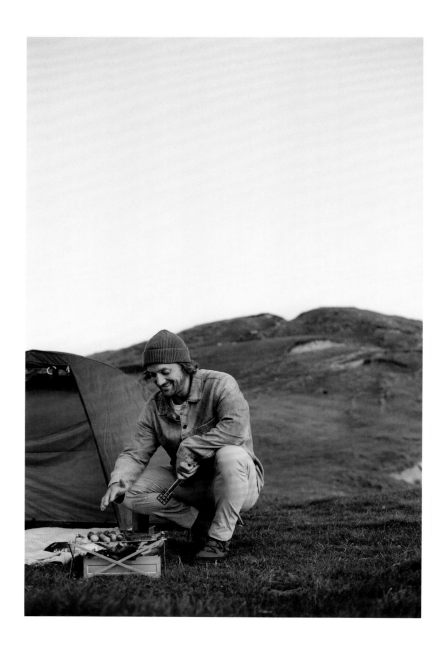

A night in the wild

If you really want to ramp up your outdoor experience, spend a night 'wild camping' – under the stars in nature, away from light pollution and the noise of the city. There is nothing quite like it for giving you that sense of total freedom.

When I sleep outside, I find it is like pressing the reset button on life. There are few other times – with the exception of surfing – that I feel so present, so alive and so at one with Mother Nature.

Why is it so rewarding?

- **You are outside.** For a long time. Properly at one with nature. And we already know the massive benefits that this brings to our mental and physical health.
- **You can only take the bare essentials.** Not carrying loads of clutter really emphasizes the break from nine-to-five life.
- **It feels like a total escape from the normal;** you have the freedom to find your own adventures, without limits.
- **It challenges you.** Chances are, you are way outside your comfort zone. You have to work out how to cook, where to sleep – and, in fact, how to sleep at all with sometimes-unnerving noises around you.
- **It makes you live in the present:** you need to concentrate on not getting cold/wet/starving/eaten alive by bugs, or accidentally bivvying in a bog.
- **You get to be outside in the evening and at dawn,** when everyone else is heading home or sleeping in their beds, back in civilization. Seeing the dawn from your 'bed' is an awe-inspiring experience that should be on everyone's checklist.
- **It's completely free!**

If the idea freaks you out a bit, start easy by camping in your back garden. Pitch a tent if you like, but diehard wild campers prefer to take just a bivvy bag (a waterproof bag you can snuggle down in, away from the elements) so they are truly sleeping under the stars. Obviously the weather will dictate how well that turns out . . .

You could then progress to a local woodland or wild space, or travel further afield to a national park. Check before you go that wild camping is allowed in that area, or book in with a campsite or friendly farmer.

Whether you go alone or with friends is up to you. However, there is extra power in a solo wilderness experience. Quality alone time allows thoughts to surface that you have maybe buried for a while, and gives you the chance to clarify your inner feelings, hopes and dreams. I find it gives me time and space to step back, reflect and evaluate my life. Are there new goals I want to set myself? Am I being productive? What is and isn't working in my life right now? It's almost like an outdoor life audit (see p. 138).

Being on your own outside at night is also a bigger adventure and is a way of challenging yourself. Research has found that a solo overnight wilderness trip gave people more confidence in themselves and made them feel more able to cope. It also gave them a sense of perspective and an appreciation of life – together with a sense of freedom, increased well-being, and an escape from the normal routine.

Other studies have found that solitary reflection enriches us physically, mentally and emotionally. It encourages reorganization of life priorities, helps you become more attuned to the important things, and increases your appreciation of silence and reflection.

A few things to remember before you set off:
- **Wild camping is legal in Scotland,** but it's technically an offence in England and Wales unless you get the landowner's permission. Some national parks do welcome wild camping, but always check before you go.
- **Wherever you camp,** it's important to think carefully about your impact. Always leave the site exactly as you found it, respect water sources, carry

home all your litter and avoid trampling sensitive habitats.

- **Make sure you know the route** that you're taking. Use an Ordnance Survey map so you can plot your journey and be aware of your surroundings.
- **Remember to always plan ahead,** and aim to get to your destination before sunset so that you have enough time to scope out your spot.
- **Always have a plan B,** and somewhere you can get to easily and safely at any point.

Mum's harvest hotpot

DINNER

Serves 4–6

I remember a classic Yorkshire hotpot was a staple after a rugby game in the clubhouse, but my mum always knew how to jazz it up and put her own veggie spin on it. My version has turned into a combination of both of them: it warms your insides, it's super-filling and it tastes epic.

2 tbsp olive oil
1 onion, diced
2 medium carrots, diced
2 leeks, sliced
3 stalks celery, diced
3 garlic cloves, finely chopped
2 heaped tsp paprika
2 tbsp tomato puree
1.2 litres vegetable stock
1 x 400g can chopped tomatoes
½ small bunch thyme
3 rosemary sprigs, roughly
    chopped
2 bay leaves
500g potatoes, cut into
    2.5-cm chunks
200g soup and broth mix (lentils
    and pulses)
2 red peppers, cut into
    2.5-cm chunks
handful flat-leaf parsley,
    roughly chopped

Heat a large casserole dish over a high heat. When hot, add the olive oil, onion and carrots and sauté for 3–4 minutes. Next add the leeks, celery and garlic, and cook for a further 5 minutes, or until all the vegetables have softened.

Stir in the paprika and tomato puree, and let it cook for a couple of minutes. Next add the stock, tomatoes and herbs, and bring up to a simmer. Add the potatoes and soup mix, and simmer gently with the lid on for 20 minutes, stirring occasionally.

Remove the lid and add the peppers, then cook for a further 10 minutes with the lid on. Season with salt and pepper to taste. Stir in the flat-leaf parsley and ladle into bowls. Serve with buttered crusty granary bread.

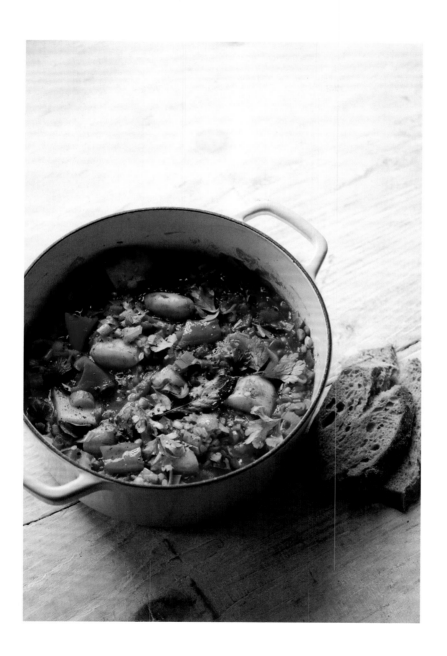

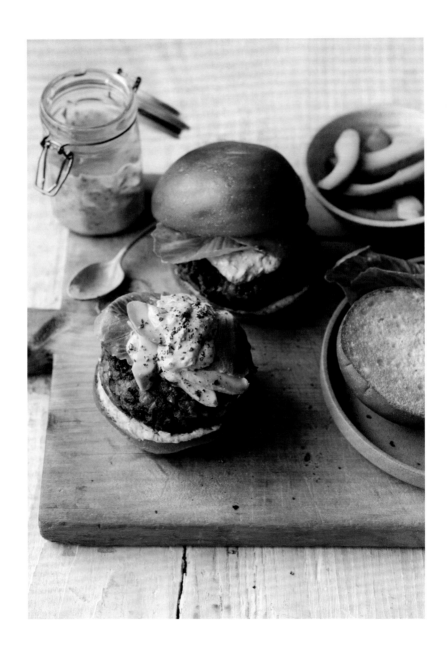

Sweet potato and bean burgers

DINNER

Makes 4

I have to thank the lady at the Bali burger shack for this one. When I was doing my yoga teacher training out there, my evening ritual was a feast at this veggie restaurant, often I'd get the beach burger with all the trimmings. This is my version of that mega-tasty dish. Pair with your choice of fries on the side.

2 large sweet potatoes
2 tbsp olive oil
1 large onion, finely chopped
2 garlic cloves, finely chopped
2 tsp hot smoked paprika
2 tsp ground cumin
½ tsp ground chilli powder
2 x 400g cans black beans,
    drained and rinsed
1 tsp dried oregano
50g panko breadcrumbs
50g roasted almonds,
    finely chopped

Chipotle sour cream
150g sour cream (or
    vegan mayo)
30g chipotle paste
juice of ½ lime
2 tbsp fresh coriander,
    finely chopped

To serve
4 wholemeal burger buns
2 ripe avocados
lettuce leaves or spinach

Preheat the oven to 200°C/180°C fan/Gas Mark 6.

Prick the sweet potatoes with a fork, and place onto a tray. Put into the oven for 30 minutes.

Meanwhile, put a large frying pan over a high heat. Pour in half the olive oil, then add the onion and sauté until softened. Reduce the heat a little and stir in the garlic for 1 minute, then add the spices and stir well. Add the black beans and oregano and remove from the heat. Using a potato masher, mash up the bean mix a little. You want them to be mashed but still retain some texture.

When the sweet potatoes are cooked, remove from the oven and leave to cool slightly. Cut them in half lengthways and scoop out the flesh into a large bowl. Mash the sweet potato and add the mashed bean mixture, breadcrumbs and almonds. Mix everything well, season with salt and pepper then divide into four portions and flatten into patties. Place the patties on a tray and leave in the fridge for an hour.

Mix everything for the chipotle sour cream and set aside.

Put the rest of the olive oil into a large non-stick frying pan over a high heat. When hot, add the patties and cook for 3–4 minutes on each side. Toast the burger-bun halves under the grill, and set aside until needed.

Assemble in your preferred order and get eating!

Veggie shepherd's pie

DINNER

A massive childhood favourite – I'd actually go over to my mate's place after school because his mum made a huge shepherd's pie and we could fill our plates. Then it was back to my house for lasagne. Thanks to the epic mums for giving me these gifts for life! This dish never gets old, and never fails to hit the spot.

1.5kg mixed root veg (I use sweet potato, swede and potato)
1 tbsp thyme leaves
2 sprigs rosemary, finely chopped
2 tbsp olive oil
1 onion, diced
2 medium carrots, diced
4 stalks celery, diced
3 garlic cloves, finely chopped
1 large courgette, diced
200g mushrooms, roughly chopped
1 tbsp thyme
1 tbsp fresh sage, finely chopped
400ml veg stock
1 x 400g can chopped tomatoes
2 x 400g cans lentils, drained (green or beluga)
1 x 400g can mixed beans, drained
200g savoy cabbage, chopped
40g butter
3 tbsp milk
1 large handful grated cheese
1–2 tbsp pumpkin seeds

To serve
salad leaves of choice

You'll need a rectangular baking dish that's about 33 x 23cm, and 5–8cm deep.

Preheat the oven to 170°C/150°C fan/Gas Mark 3.

Peel and cut the root veg into 2.5-cm chunks. Put them onto two lined oven trays. Sprinkle with thyme and rosemary, and season well with salt and pepper. Drizzle with half the olive oil and mix well, so everything is coated. Place in the oven for 40 minutes, or until tender. Remove from the oven and increase the heat to 220°C/200°C fan/Gas Mark 7.

While the veg is cooking, add the remaining oil to a large non-stick casserole pan and place over a high heat. Add the onion and carrots and sauté for 4 minutes before adding the celery and garlic. Cook for a further 2 minutes before adding the courgette, mushrooms, herbs, stock and tomatoes. Bring up to a simmer and cook for 10 minutes, then add the lentils, beans and cabbage. Cook for 5 minutes more, season to taste, and then spoon into the baking dish.

Once it's out of the oven, transfer the roast veg to a large bowl. Add the butter and milk and mash well with a potato masher. Spoon the mash over the lentil mixture. Sprinkle with grated cheese and pumpkin seeds and place in the oven for 20 minutes, or until the cheese has melted and browned. Remove and serve with some salad while it's HOT!

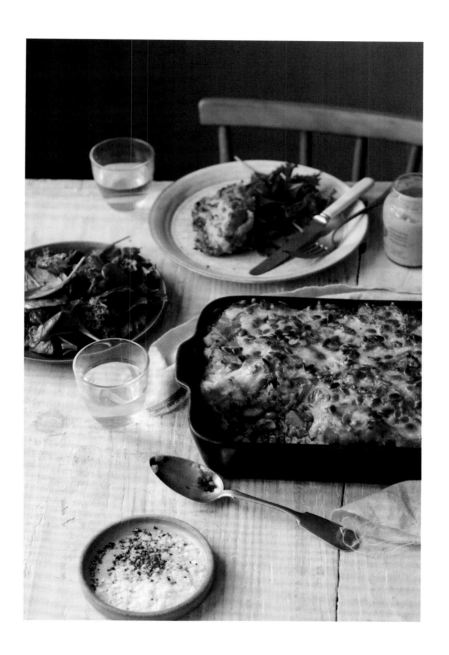

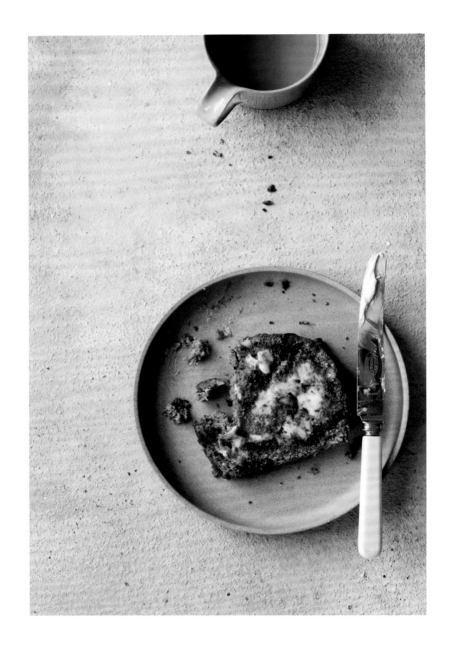

Loaded banana bread

SNACKS

Serves 8

This is so full of goodness – it can be super-filling and could almost make a meal per slice! It's my favourite accompaniment to tea and post-training snack, but it's basically an essential bit of baking for any occasion in my eyes.

2 large free-range eggs
100g light muscovado sugar
3 medium overripe bananas,
   mashed well
150ml coconut oil, melted
1 tsp vanilla extract
50ml oat milk
250g wholemeal
   self-raising flour
2 tsp baking powder
½ tsp salt
1 tsp ground cinnamon
½ tsp ground cardamom
1 tbsp chia seeds
100g toasted pecans, chopped
50g toasted pumpkin seeds
120g dark chocolate chips

To serve
butter, or nut butter of choice

Preheat the oven to 190°C/170°C fan/Gas Mark 5.

Put the eggs and muscovado sugar into the bowl of a stand mixer and whisk for 5–8 minutes, or until thick, pale and creamy. Alternatively, you can do this with a hand mixer.

Add the bananas to the bowl, along with the melted coconut oil, vanilla and oat milk. Mix gently until incorporated. Add the flour, baking powder, salt, spices and chia seeds to the bowl, and mix with a rubber spatula until smooth. Stir in the pecans, pumpkin seeds and chocolate chips.

Line a 900-gram loaf tin with greaseproof paper. Spoon the batter into the tin, then place it in the preheated oven for 50 minutes–1 hour. Test by inserting a skewer into the middle of the cake – if it comes out clean, it's cooked.

Leave to cool in the tin for 5 minutes. Then remove from the tin and leave to cool on a wire rack before enjoying with your choice of butter.

Cupboard staples

These are the key items that I always have, so that when I don't have time to plan my meals I can whip up something delicious. So if you invest in these items and always have veggies in, you'll be able to make the most of my recipes.

Agave/maple syrup – These can be used interchangeably, for sweetness.

Alfalfa sprouts – These can be swapped out for cress or any other sprout, and if you have kids these are super-fun and easy to grow at home with them!

Breakfast superfood mix – I use crushed almonds (toasted in the oven for a few minutes until browned), cacao nibs and sunflower, pumpkin, chia and sesame seeds.

Chia seeds – These are a great addition to smoothies and breakfasts, and are packed full of essential nutrients.

Furikake – This is a mix made with dried seaweed and sesame seeds, and is a staple of

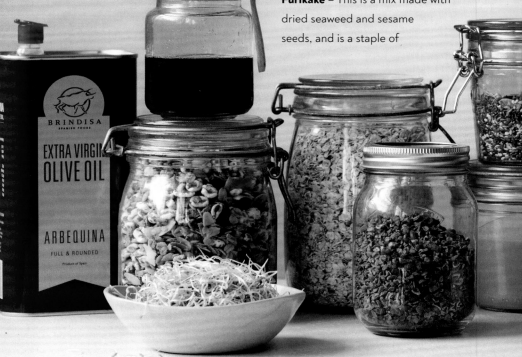

Japanese cooking. You can also use sesame seeds as an alternative.

Kaffir lime leaves – These are ideal for a tasty Asian flavour, but you can always use lime zest if you can't get hold of them (I'd say use the zest of half a lime in place of two leaves).

Kimchi – This is fermented cabbage, way tastier than it sounds and full of microorganisms that boost your immune system and fight inflammation. It's in most large supermarkets but I love that every batch I make is a bit different.

Nuts – I like pecans, cashews, pistachios and almonds.

Porridge oats – Something I could never live without. Porridge is part of my heritage and always hits the spot.

Savoury seed mix – I always have a jar of mixed seeds that have been toasted in a frying pan with a splash of soy. These add a nice crunch to lots of dishes. I use sunflower, pumpkin, sesame and flax seeds, but you can create your own mix.

Shaoxing – This is a classic ingredient in Chinese cuisine and creates a really authentic flavour, but if you can't get hold of it then any rice wine will do.

Soy sauce – I use light soy sauce in my recipes but feel free to use your favourite kind.

Tahini – This is essential for making creamy hummus. It's also a really tasty base for dressings.

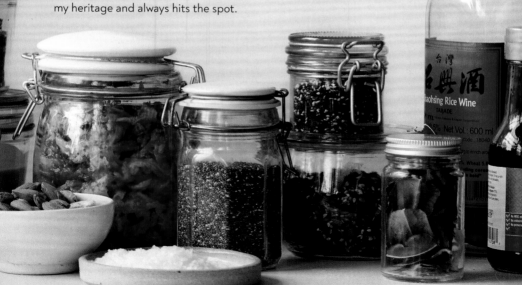

Further reading and resources

I have been inspired by so many ground-breaking, thoughtful and inspiring people – here are some of their books, podcasts and websites, if you want to check out their work and deepen your understanding of the practices I feature in this book.

BREATHWORK

Donna Farhi, *The Breathing Book: Vitality and Good Health through Essential Breath Work* (Holt Paperbacks, 1996). This is a great guide to yoga breathing.

Patrick McKeown, *Buteyko Clinic Method* (with CD and DVD) (OxyAt Books, 2019).

Patrick McKeown, *The Oxygen Advantage: The Simple, Scientifically Proven Breathing Technique That Will Revolutionise Your Health and Fitness* (Piatkus, 2015), https://oxygenadvantage.com.

James Nestor, *Breath: The New Science of a Lost Art* (Penguin, 2020).

Rob Wilson, *weMove* podcast, episode 3, 'Art of Breath', https://wemove.world/podcasts/2018/6/1/mover-rob-wilson-art-of-breath.

Shift (https://shiftadapt.com) – an organization founded by Brian Mackenzie.

YOGA

I rarely practise traditional yoga these days, but I do incorporate the techniques into my movement and breathwork, and was inspired by my original yoga teachers Eoin Finn (see https://blissology.com for videos and podcasts) and Zephyr Wildman (@zephyrwildman on Instagram; https://zephyryoga.com for podcasts and class details).

PERFORMANCE AND MINDSET

Ant Middleton, *The Fear Bubble: Harness Fear and Live Without Limits* (HarperCollins, 2020).

Ant Middleton, *First Man In: Leading from the Front* (HarperCollins, 2019).

Timothy Ferriss, *The 4-Hour Work Week: Escape the 9-5, Live Anywhere and Join the New Rich* (Vermilion, 2011).

Logan Gelbrich, *Going Right: A Logical Justification for Pursuing Your Dreams* (Gelbrich Development, 2019). You can also find him on Instagram as @functionalcoach.

XPT (Extreme Performance Training) (www.xptlife.com) – founded by surfer Laird

Hamilton (https://www.lairdhamilton.com) and his partner, the athlete Gabby Reece.

NATURE

George Monbiot, *Feral: Rewilding the Land, Sea and Human Life* (Penguin, 2014).

NUTRITION

Jamie Oliver was the first chef who got me to play and freestyle in the kitchen (https://www.jamieoliver.com).

More recently I have been inspired by Bettina Campolucci Bordi (https://www.bettinaskitchen.com; or @bettinas_kitchen on Instagram) and her book *Happy Food: Fast, Fresh, Simple Vegan* (Hardie Grant, 2018).

Also David and Stephen Flynn from The Happy Pear (https://thehappypear.ie) and their books *The Happy Pear: Healthy, Easy, Delicious Food to Change Your Life* (Penguin Ireland, 2014) and *The World of the Happy Pear* (Penguin Ireland, 2016).

HEALTH

Megan Rossi, *The Gut Health Doctor, Eat Yourself Healthy: An Easy-To-Digest Guide to Health and Happiness from the Inside Out* (Penguin Life, 2019).

Matthew Walker, *Why We Sleep: The New Science of Sleep and Dreams* (Penguin, 2017).

INSPIRATIONAL PODCASTS

Fearne Cotton's *Happy Place* podcast, https://www.officialfearnecotton.com/news/2018/2/26/happy-place-podcast.

The *Rich Roll* Podcast, https://www.richroll.com/category/podcast – the ultra-endurance athlete has been producing chart-topping podcasts since 2013.

Tony Robbins, https://www.tonyrobbins.com/podcasts – discusses useful strategies for achieving your goals.

weMove, https://wemove.world/podcasts – a huge variety of episodes on health and well-being.

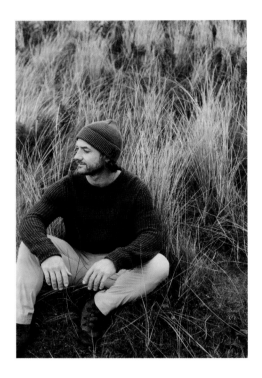

Acknowledgements

Creating this book has been a wild and powerful journey. It would not have been possible without the help, guidance and support from the awesome crew at Penguin. Thanks Emily for believing in me and this book idea from the start. Then the dream team that brought it all together, kept the vibe high and made it a lot of fun: Saffron and Amy you are absolute legends. Issy's camera mastery, Nicole's help getting creative in the kitchen, Rachel's patience following me around for months trying to make sense of all my stories, and Tamara for all your love. I appreciate you all.

Index

Recipe index